Water, Sanitation and Hygiene in Humanitarian Contexts

Praise for this book

'WASH (Water, Sanitation and Hygiene) is a crucial component of humanitarian response. This book is a very useful compilation of lessons learned from a range of highly experienced and qualified practitioners in the field, compiled by Richard Carter, one of the most respected experts. It also provides recommendations for how WASH in emergencies can be improved, and highlights some major gaps, such as the transition from emergency response to longer term recovery. It will be of interest to emergency WASH practitioners and those involved (or preparing to be involved) in humanitarian action.

Bobby Lambert, co-author of Engineering in Emergencies and consultant in humanitarian action

'Essential reading! A mine of useful and useable information for anyone working within the complexity of disaster situations. Richard Carter and his colleagues bring rich experiences and insights concerning water, sanitation and hygiene in crisis conditions to both general and experienced readers.'

Ian Davis is Visiting Professor in Disaster Risk Management in Copenhagen, Lund, Kyoto and Oxford Brookes Universities

'Water, Sanitation and Hygiene in Humanitarian Contexts is absolutely right at the heart of the main water, hygiene and sanitation challenges in emergencies.'

Jean-Francois Fesselet, WatSan unit Coordinator, MSF

Water, Sanitation and Hygiene in Humanitarian Contexts
Reflections on current practice

Edited by Richard C. Carter

KEY WRITINGS ON WASH IN
INTERNATIONAL DEVELOPMENT

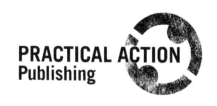

Practical Action Publishing Ltd
The Schumacher Centre,
Bourton on Dunsmore, Rugby,
Warwickshire, CV23 9QZ, UK
www.practicalactionpublishing.org

© Practical Action Publishing, 2015

All the chapters in this book, except for chapters 1 and 4, were first published as articles in *Waterlines: an international journal of water, sanitation and waste*.

The right of the editor to be identified as author of the editorial material and of the contributors for their individual chapters have been asserted under sections 77 and 78 of the Copyright Designs and Patents Act 1988.

All rights reserved. No part of this publication may be reprinted or reproduced or utilized in any form or by any electronic, mechanical, or other means, now known or hereafter invented, including photocopying and recording, or in any information storage or retrieval system, without the written permission of the publishers.

Product or corporate names may be trademarks or registered trademarks, and are used only for identification and explanation without intent to infringe.

A catalogue record for this book is available from the British Library.
A catalogue record for this book has been requested from the Library of Congress.

ISBN 978-1-85339-883-4 Hardback
ISBN 978-1-85339-884-1 Paperback
ISBN 978-1-78044-883-1 Library Ebook
ISBN 978-1-78044-884-8 Ebook

Citation: Carter, Richard C. (ed.) (2015) Water, *Sanitation and Hygiene in Humanitarian Contexts: Reflections on current practice*, Rugby, UK: Practical Action Publishing, <http://dx.doi.org/ 9781780448831 >

Since 1974, Practical Action Publishing has published and disseminated books and information in support of international development work throughout the world. Practical Action Publishing is a trading name of Practical Action Publishing Ltd (Company Reg. No. 1159018), the wholly owned publishing company of Practical Action. Practical Action Publishing trades only in support of its parent charity objectives and any profits are covenanted back to Practical Action (Charity Reg. No. 247257, Group VAT Registration No. 880 9924 76).

The views and opinions in this publication are those of the author and do not represent those of Practical Action Publishing Ltd or its parent charity Practical Action. Reasonable efforts have been made to publish reliable data and information, but the authors and publisher cannot assume responsibility for the validity of all materials or for the consequences of their use.

Cover design by Practical Action Publishing
Typeset by Allzone Digital
Printed in the United Kingdom

FSC

Contents

1. Introduction: Water, sanitation and hygiene in humanitarian contexts ... 1
   Richard C. Carter

2. Point-of-use water treatment in emergency response ... 13
   Daniele Lantagne and Thomas Clasen

3. Water, sanitation, and hygiene in emergencies: summary review and recommendations for further research ... 35
   Joe Brown, Sue Cavill, Oliver Cumming and Aurelie Jeandron

4. Water and wastes in the context of the West African Ebola outbreak: turning uncertain science into pragmatic guidance in Sierra Leone ... 53
   Richard C. Carter, J. Peter Dumble, St John Day, and Michael Cowing

5. Menstrual hygiene management in humanitarian emergencies: gaps and recommendations ... 63
   Marni Sommer

6. Bulk water treatment unit performance: for the cameras or the community? ... 83
   Richard Luff and Caetano Dorea

7. Innovative designs and approaches in sanitation when responding to challenging and complex humanitarian contexts in urban areas ... 97
   Andy Bastable and Jenny Lamb

8. Biodegradable bags as emergency sanitation in urban settings: the field experience ... 113
   Francesca Coloni, Rafael van den Bergh, Federico Sittaro, Stephanie Giandonato, Geneviève Loots and Peter Maes

9. Urban armed conflicts and water services ... 123
   Jean-François Pinera

10. Sanitation for all! Free of cost in emergencies ... 139
    Marco Visser

11. Conclusions ... 143
    Richard C. Carter

http://dx.doi.org/10.3362/9781780448831.000

About the editor

Richard Carter (richard@richard-carter.org) has worked in the science, engineering and management of water and sanitation since 1975. He has undertaken assignments in numerous countries in sub-Saharan Africa and Asia, and published widely. From a base in academia and consultancy, he has worked with and for national Governments, bilateral and multilateral agencies and INGOs, always with a primary focus on low-income countries and fragile states. He has been Technical Editor and Editor of *Waterlines* journal since 2002. Since 2012 he undertakes all his work through his own consultancy firm (www.richard-carter.org).

CHAPTER 1
Introduction: Water, sanitation and hygiene in humanitarian contexts

Richard C. Carter

Abstract

This introductory chapter explains the origins, scope and intended readership of Water, Sanitation and Hygiene in Humanitarian Contexts. *It describes the human impacts of emergencies and disasters, briefly discusses some of the terms used in humanitarian work, and examines the diversity of types of emergency and disaster. The introduction then moves on to some of the specifics of water, sanitation and hygiene – WASH – in emergencies, referring extensively to the Sphere Handbook,* Humanitarian Charter and Minimum Standards in Humanitarian Response. *The final sections of the introduction touch on the challenges of transitioning from emergency to post-emergency, when resources and institutional capacity may be very different to the acute phase of the emergency. Lastly, the individual chapters of the book are summarized and suggestions are made as to how the book can most usefully be read.*

In 2011, the world saw a massive earthquake, tsunami and nuclear meltdown in Japan; devastating drought in East Africa; extreme and costly floods in Thailand; and a damaging but under-reported typhoon in the Philippines. Since that time there has been a seemingly relentless unfolding of natural disasters – earthquakes, storms, floods and droughts – and still unresolved fighting in Central African Republic, South Sudan and Syria. At the time of writing, we are eight months into the world's worst Ebola outbreak in West Africa. All these examples, and many others, have implications for water and sanitation services.

The impact of emergencies and disasters is inevitably greater in what have come to be called 'fragile states' than in those which by virtue of effective government, strong institutions and wealthier economies have greater resilience to such events. In fragile states, periods of relative stability, in which development efforts make some progress, are often punctuated by crises which may have long-lasting impacts. Effective long-term development is the best form of disaster-risk reduction, and good governance and strong institutions represent the best form of disaster preparedness.

All of these crises, disasters or emergencies – choose your term – profoundly affect individual human beings, their families, their communities, the surrounding populations, and the nations in which these events take place. They all demand rapid and effective response to physical need – of which water and sanitation is one part – and longer-term recovery and reconstruction.

This book is not and cannot be a comprehensive treatise on disaster response (let alone disaster preparedness or post-disaster recovery). Rather it sets out a number of very down-to-earth issues and actions which have been addressed and undertaken by practitioner organizations in recent years. The individual contributions in the chapters which follow this scene-setting introduction fit within wider social, economic and political contexts. They address particular aspects of WASH – water, sanitation and hygiene – and taken together they give a useful flavour of the thinking, experimentation and reflection of those who are constantly striving for greater effectiveness in humanitarian emergency response.

Who the book is for

This book is for those whose work regularly involves them in providing WASH in emergencies, but it should also be of interest to those who are mainly involved in long-term development, from WASH and other sectors. It will be of value to those studying for technical and professional qualifications in WASH and in disaster management. It demonstrates the wide range of issues which WASH professionals have to address as they attempt to respond to emergencies.

Humanitarian disasters and emergencies

Neither the phrase 'humanitarian emergency', nor the more pithy reference to a 'disaster', do justice to the effects caused by such events. Imagine for some moments what happens when an emergency unfolds, when a sudden flood or earthquake hits, when a drought sets in, or when society falls apart during conflict.

The 'emergency' can happen either gradually (in the case of slow-onset droughts and famines) or suddenly (rapid-onset earthquakes and floods). Individuals and families lose their homes, their possessions, and, in some cases, their lives or those of loved ones. The number of deaths is what hits the news headlines and is the popular, if blunt, measure of the severity of the emergency. 'Thousands killed in disaster' shocks newspaper readers, but fails to reflect the reality for those who live on. For every death there are many times as many who survive, affected physically, mentally, and socially.

Those who survive may become 'displaced': no longer able to live in the places they once called home. If they cross national borders, they become refugees. They may reach the relative safety of family elsewhere, of towns or cities which they do not know, or of a hastily constructed 'camp'. Camps for internally displaced persons (IDPs) or refugees may take the form of tented cities or accommodation built in local styles and materials, but for their residents they represent more than a mere physical displacement. People are dislocated physically, socially and mentally. They are dislocated, along with all their pre-existing health needs and infirmities, and with all their individual and family frailties and strengths. Livings are disrupted, and those with least in reserve are naturally hardest hit. Social networks are upset as whole communities are displaced. People suffer loss, shock, stress and uncertainty.

These are some of the realities for those who have survived death and been displaced from their homes by the emergency. There are other emergencies, however, which do not cause displacement – sometimes it can be precisely the opposite. As I write this, the Ebola outbreak in Guinea, Sierra Leone and Liberia is continuing. For those affected, 'lock-down' – prevention of movement and interaction – is the pattern, rather than escape. Yet the effects for those surviving are similar – livings are disrupted, and uncertainty, suspicion, and fear abound.

Every emergency is different in its details, despite some common features across certain categories. It may be that the apparently increasing diversity of emergencies reflects our increasing understanding of their nuances, and it is certainly true that large-scale demographic changes and the evolving nature of armed conflict are resulting in more people being affected by a wider range of types of emergency than ever before. The world is becoming more complex and unpredictable.

Disasters and emergencies not only affect those they kill and those who are left behind, but the communities, societies and nations where displaced people end up. They affect national economies, sometimes retarding investment and development for many years. In the case of war or other large-scale armed conflict, it is uncommon for visible progress to be seen in the processes of healing, renewal and restoration of confidence and security until a decade or more has passed.

Those affected by a disaster may need immediate fundamentals: shelter, food, water and sanitation, clothing and household goods; they may need health services and education – the children affected by the civil war in Syria have missed out on much schooling, and the closure of schools in Sierra Leone in response to Ebola has robbed children of a full year of education. This book addresses some aspects of WASH, but it is important to set these in the wider context of need.

Definitions and diversity

As with all fields of endeavour, there is a body of jargon which we need to deal with in the interests of clear communication. First, the word 'humanitarian' itself, which, according to the dictionary, means 'concerned with or seeking to improve human welfare'. In the present context, however, the word is used to refer to extraordinary events which have affected human beings, and which require urgent action – disasters or emergencies. This is in contrast to the concern for improving human welfare which is embodied in long-term sustainable development work.

According to ReliefWeb (2008) a **disaster** is 'a serious disruption of the functioning of a community or a society causing widespread human, material, economic or environmental losses which exceed the ability of the affected community or society to cope using its own resources'. An **emergency** is 'a sudden and usually unforeseen event that calls for immediate measures to minimize its adverse consequences'. The two terms are often used interchangeably, although some argue that a disaster is larger in scale than many emergencies; a local emergency may or may not develop into a full-blown disaster. Some put emergencies, disasters and catastrophes on a sliding scale of increasing severity. A **crisis** – 'a time of extreme difficulty or danger' – or an emergency may develop into a disaster.

Emergencies and disasters have many root causes and triggers. Various categorizations exist, with the primary categories being **natural disasters** (e.g. earthquake, storm, flood, drought, epidemic), **technological disasters** (various kinds of accidents) and **'complex humanitarian emergencies'** – those having multiple causes and in which violence, insecurity and breakdown of law and order often compound the difficulties faced by those who are affected. Table 1.1 summarises these categories, according to the International Federation of Red Cross and Red Crescent Societies. As well as the categories of disaster listed, a number of aggravating factors are highlighted – interestingly with no reference to general population growth, which surely accounts for much of the growth in disasters over recent years.

Table 1.1 Categories of humanitarian disaster (IFRC, 2014)

Category	Sub-category	Examples
Natural	Geophysical	Earthquakes, landslides, tsunamis, volcanic eruptions
	Hydrological	Avalanches, floods
	Climatological	Extreme temperatures, drought, wildfires
	Meteorological	Cyclones, storm surges
	Biological	Disease epidemics, insect/animal plagues
Technological	Industrial accidents	Release of chemicals or radioactivity into the environment
	Transport accidents	Air crash, road crash
Complex emergencies/ conflicts	War/conflict	Civil strife, cross-border fighting
	Famine	Chronic and acute food insecurity
Aggravating factors	Climate change	
	Unplanned urbanization	
	Under-development/ poverty	
	Threat of pandemics	

Disasters result when people live in hazardous situations (e.g. in floodplains or seismically active zones), an event occurs (flood or earthquake in the examples given), the population is vulnerable (e.g. as a result of its physical location or its poverty) and its capacity to cope is limited (e.g. because of limited resources or weak institutions).

Wherever and however a natural or man-made disaster affects people, basic services, including those of water and sanitation, may be disrupted. Prolonged droughts may reduce stocks of water; flooding and geophysical disasters (such as earthquakes and volcanic eruptions) may damage water supply and sanitation infrastructure; industrial accidents may pollute water resources; any form of human displacement may reduce people's access to services.

Disruption of water and sanitation services creates problems for those affected. But WASH actions also form part of the solution – when done well, they can help to safeguard health – especially by controlling outbreaks of water-related diseases such as cholera – and preserve dignity and well-being at a time when all of these are in short supply.

The importance of WASH in emergencies and disasters

Emergencies and disasters affect WASH services and practices by damaging existing infrastructure or by separating displaced populations from the services which they had enjoyed. In the case of displacement, host populations are also affected, as greater demands are placed on their services. Those who reach the relative safety of IDP and refugee camps may be there for many years or even decades before repatriation.

The *Humanitarian Charter and Minimum Standards in Disaster Response* (known in short as the Sphere Handbook, 2011) sets out standards and guidance in relation to four fundamentals, of which WASH is the first. The others are Food Security and Nutrition, Shelter, Settlement and Non-Food Items, and Health Action.

The Handbook explains why WASH is so important in disasters: 'Water and sanitation are critical determinants for survival in the initial stages of a disaster. People affected by disasters are generally much more susceptible to illness and death from disease, which to a large extent are related to inadequate sanitation, inadequate water supplies and inability to maintain good hygiene. The most significant of these diseases are diarrhoeal and infectious diseases transmitted by the faeco-oral route. Other water- and sanitation-related diseases include those carried by vectors associated with solid waste and water.'

The maintenance of good health is justifiably one of the most important considerations for doing WASH in emergencies and disasters. However, just as in long-term development situations, there are several other reasons for doing WASH, and doing it well. Adequate water supply is a basic need for drinking and cooking, laundry, personal and home hygiene. Safe and private latrines or toilets are necessary because the opportunity to practice good hygiene is not just the means of preserving health, but a matter of human dignity.

The various components of WASH each have aspects which are common to emergencies and to non-emergency situations; and they each have aspects which are particular to emergencies.

Water supply

Standards of access, quantity and quality of water supply in emergencies have much in common with similar considerations in the absence of an emergency. An important difference, however, is that unlike the case of rural water supply more generally – in which protected, 'improved' water sources are used – emergency water supply is always treated. Water provided for potable uses is nearly always chlorinated, and consequently one of the tests used for water supplied in emergencies is the chlorine residual.

Water supplied in emergencies is usually provided free-of-charge to the consumers – a significant difference from normal practice in urban and rural water supply generally. This has important implications post-emergency.

High standard treatment of water, and non-payment for water, are generally true in the acute phase of an emergency, but many IDP and refugee camps last for years or even decades. Further reference is made below to the transition from emergency to post-emergency measures.

Sanitation

The term 'sanitation', throughout the Sphere Handbook, refers to excreta disposal, vector control, solid waste disposal and drainage. This broad definition is just as appropriate to non-emergency situations as to emergencies. Defining sanitation simply in terms of excreta disposal is too narrow a point of view, in general, and in emergencies.

The purpose of sanitation in the broad sense is to keep the environment in which people live free of hazardous wastes, and to reduce disease transmission by insect and animal vectors.

The Sphere Handbook explains the importance of disease vectors: 'A vector is a disease-carrying agent and vector-borne diseases are a major cause of sickness and death in many disaster situations. Mosquitoes are the vector responsible for malaria transmission, which is one of the leading causes of morbidity and mortality. Mosquitoes also transmit other diseases, such as yellow fever, dengue and haemorrhagic fever. Non-biting or synanthropic flies, such as the house fly, the blow fly and the flesh fly, play an important role in the transmission of diarrhoeal disease. Biting flies, bedbugs and fleas are a painful nuisance and in some cases transmit significant diseases such as murine typhus, scabies and plague. Ticks transmit relapsing fever, while human body lice transmit typhus and relapsing fever. Rats and mice can transmit diseases, such as leptospirosis and salmonellosis, and can be hosts for other vectors, e.g. fleas, which may transmit Lassa fever, plague and other infections.'

Control of disease vectors is especially important in densely populated IDP and refugee camps, as in urban areas generally. A number of different measures may need to be taken to control vectors; at the level of the individual, the dwelling and the wider environment. As is the case with hygiene, knowledge and understanding are good starting points, but these are not necessarily sufficient to bring about action or changed behaviours.

Hygiene promotion

The Sphere Handbook describes hygiene promotion as 'a planned, systematic approach to enable people to take action to prevent and/or mitigate water, sanitation and hygiene-related diseases.' This section of the handbook identifies three key factors which enable people to take action:

1. a mutual sharing of information and knowledge;
2. the mobilization of affected communities; and
3. the provision of essential materials and facilities.

The first and third of these are necessary but not sufficient. For hygiene promotion to be planned and systematic, the second, 'mobilization', must be based on sound understanding of the existing practices of the affected populations, of the factors which motivate those people to practice good hygiene and sanitation, and on the psychology of behaviour and habit.

In emergencies and more generally, hygiene promotion suffers the irony of being simultaneously of greatest importance to health and yet generally the least systematically undertaken. The Sphere Handbook's use of the words 'planned, systematic' to describe hygiene promotion is both highly pertinent and also highly aspirational.

The changing nature of emergencies and disasters

While it may have been the case in the past that most disasters were caused by the impact of natural events on largely rural populations, that situation is certainly no longer true. Global population – and especially the populations of low-income and fragile states – is still growing. Habitation is urbanizing. Industries are developing. The nature of conflicts and the politics which surround them are changing. Future emergencies and disasters may be more urban in nature, more complex, and more political.

These and other trends will demand a wider range of skills in emergency WASH personnel than even now. WASH in emergencies cannot be simply a technical response to a physical need: the context is changing.

One aspect of the changing context is the blurring of lines between traditional WASH-in-emergency actors (the WASH Cluster system, in which humanitarian agencies from the United Nations and INGO sectors collaborate) and new actors – development organizations getting involved in emergency response. Collaboration between these different actors is to be welcomed, but any hint of amateurism – well-meaning but ill-informed and unprofessional intervention – is most certainly not.

The end of the emergency

Immediate response to an emergency is relatively short-lived. The age-old problem of how emergency responses should evolve into solutions which will serve affected populations for many years or even decades remains. Once media attention moves on and funding diminishes, how will local institutions be able to modify, manage and finance the services which camp-dwellers in particular still need? How should the roles of the affected populations change over time? How should services be provided to returnees?

Post-emergency transitions

Emergencies, disasters and crises come to an end. Those endings may be as sudden or as slow as the beginnings. The people who have been directly or indirectly affected start the transition back to normality. The transition may involve returning home. It may involve coming to terms with unwelcome memories of natural or man-made events. Those events, and the ways in which they were managed, may have given people both positive and negative examples on which to model their future lives.

The return of IDPs and refugees to their lands and homes is not without challenges. The individual attitudes of returnees – often characterized by a strong sense of dependency created by the 'handout' conditions of humanitarian emergencies – make the transition to self-reliance difficult. Returnees may have been badly scarred, mentally and physically, by their experiences. The conditions to which returnees return involve those who stayed, and re-integration may be difficult for many reasons. Just as an influx of IDPs or refugees can put great pressure on host populations, so also an influx of returnees can put pressure on the communities of those who stayed, and on services – including water supply and sanitation – which now have to be shared.

From emergency response to sustainable services

The key transition from emergency response to the post-emergency setting is how services will be managed long-term. In professional emergency response, services are provided free-of-charge, and managed by external (UN or INGO) agencies. At least in the earliest days of an emergency, user participation is limited (although there are good examples of CLTS and community health clubs being used in emergency settings). Long-term, national and local institutions have to take on joint management responsibility with participating service users, and the issue of payment for services has to be addressed. Without this triumvirate of participation, joint management and credible financing, services crumble.

Summary

An emergency, disaster or crisis causes individual suffering and loss, as well as severing community ties and disrupting nations. Many such events cause physical displacement, either within the country (the situation of IDPs) or across national borders (the situation of refugees). Where displacement is involved, this affects not only those who have been displaced, but also those nations, societies, towns and villages which act as hosts to an influx of people.

Whether or not people are displaced by an emergency, it is imperative that water supply and sanitation services and the opportunities to practice good hygiene are provided. The more that the affected populations can learn to appreciate the advantages of WASH, the more likely will be their continued enjoyment of such services after the emergency is over.

However, it is probably in the transitions from emergency to post-emergency that the humanitarian and development professions still do least well. The fact that this book, while focusing on WASH in emergencies, includes very little on the transition to and management of the post-emergency situation is illustrative of that fact. WASH in development and WASH in emergencies have much in common, but there are some important differences in approach which have implications for WASH services post-emergency. WASH in the continuum from normality through emergency to post-emergency hardly exists as a field of good professional practice.

In this book

The body of the book consists of eight chapters contributed by different authors, all of whom are widely experienced in WASH, and WASH in emergencies. Each chapter brings another context, another viewpoint, and some highly practical findings, conclusions and recommendations. The following paragraphs give a flavour of each main chapter.

In Chapter 2 Daniele Lantagne and Thomas Clasen tackle the topic of point-of-use water treatment (POUWT) in emergencies. They find that POUWT can be effective particularly in small-scale (non-acute) emergencies where diarrhoea risk is high. However, the effectiveness of POUWT depends on user preferences regarding technology and (in the case of chlorination) chlorine dosage, the provision of adequate training, and the availability of stocks of materials and products. The authors also point out the importance of seeing POUWT as part of a wider safe water strategy, and further ensuring long-term access to products for sustainability.

In Chapter 3 Joe Brown and colleagues acknowledge the key role of WASH in limiting diarrhoeal outbreaks in emergencies. They argue, however, that WASH responses could be made even more effective. They highlight a number of key areas requiring further R&D, notably innovative sanitation options for difficult settings (high water table, unstable soils, urban environments); technologies for water supply for dispersed communities; approaches to promote correct and sustained use of water quality interventions; and effective hardware and software for hand-washing promotion.

In Chapter 4, Richard Carter and colleagues describe the development of guidance on the protection of water resources and on waste management in the context of the West African Ebola crisis of 2014–15. The difficulties of communicating uncertain science into a situation of extreme risk to life are set out, and some of the research needs highlighted by the crisis are outlined.

In Chapter 5 Marni Sommer draws attention to the growing attention to menstrual hygiene management (MHM) needs in emergency responses. She points out that there is insufficient documentation of the most effective and culturally appropriate responses. Her chapter begins this documentation, and highlights the remaining gaps in MHM research, practice and policy in emergencies. Marni provides six key recommendations to those who are serious about addressing this key issue in WASH services.

In Chapter 6 Richard Luff and Caetano Dorea question whether the deployment of bulk water treatment units (BWTUs), as for example in the Pakistan floods of 2010, was a cost-effective and appropriate solution, or rather a public-relations exercise. They argue that some BWTUs represent poor value for money and too complex and sophisticated an option. They call for sector-wide selection criteria for such technologies, and wider testing by manufacturers under realistic field conditions. They further conclude that household water treatment and safe storage (otherwise known as point-of-use water treatment) may be more cost-effective and flexible options in unpredictable crises.

In Chapter 7 Andy Bastable and Jenny Lamb examine a range of situations in which provision of sanitation is especially difficult – for example in urban settings, and in difficult ground conditions, where water tables are high. They review the situations in the Haiti earthquake of 2010, and floods in the Philippines and Pakistan in 2009 and 2010 respectively. Despite the difficulties inherent in such situations, and the limited range of sanitation technology available, the authors draw out valuable and positive lessons, set out a list of 13 missing technologies, and make strong recommendations to donors and agencies involved in emergency response.

In Chapter 8 Francesca Coloni and colleagues analyse field experience of the use of biodegradable bags for emergency sanitation. Their field work was based in the camps in Port-au-Prince, Haiti, following the 2010 earthquake. The authors found that while the construction and maintenance of suitable facilities for this 'technology' was undemanding, rapid acquisition of suitable bags, and the uptake of bag usage were much less satisfactory. Uptake rates of only 13% in this large-scale intervention contrast with much higher rates in another small-scale trial. The authors conclude that the approach has its place – as a stop-gap measure, and with several important caveats.

In Chapter 9 Jean-François Pinera's chapter concerns the impact of armed conflict on city and town water supply. The author examined the cases of Kabul (Afghanistan), Jaffna (Sri Lanka), Monrovia (Liberia), Béni (DRC),

Port-au-Prince (Haiti) and Grozny (Chechnya) – towns or cities ranging in population from 78,000 to 2.9 million. He describes how various aid agencies assisted, both during and after the acute phase of the fighting. He concludes that there were few examples of such partnerships resulting in the strengthening of national institutions and the achievement of sustainability. He calls for a paradigm shift in the way aid agencies interact with national institutions, involving more meaningful partnerships, a focus on sustainable and universal service, and building confidence between national institutions and external aid agencies.

In Chapter 10 Marco Visser argues that, while water supply and food are provided free in refugee camps, sanitation facilities are constructed using refugee labour and materials. He asks why, at a time when they are most exhausted or traumatized, this should be so; he urges that aid agencies should treat sanitation in the same way as food and water, and provide it for free.

How to read this book

Since the book is a collection of stand-alone contributions, as a reader you can dip in anywhere, and read the chapters in any order. In a few cases there are cross-references from one chapter to another, but I hope this will simply encourage you to read all the chapters!

About the author

Richard Carter (richard@richard-carter.org) has worked in the science, engineering and management of water and sanitation since 1975. He has undertaken assignments in numerous countries in sub-Saharan Africa and Asia, and published widely. From a base in academia and consultancy, he has worked with and for national Governments, bilateral and multilateral agencies and INGOs, always with a primary focus on low-income countries and fragile states. Since 2012 he undertakes all his work through his own consultancy firm (www.richard-carter.org).

References

IFRC (2014) *Types of disasters: Definition of hazard.* http://www.ifrc.org/en/what-we-do/disaster-management/about-disasters/definition-of-hazard/ [last accessed 5th January 2015].

ReliefWeb (2008) *Glossary of Humanitarian Terms.* http://reliefweb.int/report/world/reliefweb-glossary-humanitarian-terms [accessed 5th January 2015].

Sphere Handbook (2011) *Humanitarian Charter and Minimum Standards in Humanitarian Response.* http://www.developmentbookshelf.com/doi/book/10.3362/9781908176202 [accessed 22nd May 2015].

WASH Cluster Homepage. http://washcluster.net [accessed 5th January 2015].

CHAPTER 2

Point-of-use water treatment in emergency response

Daniele Lantagne and Thomas Clasen

Abstract

Point-of-use water treatment (PoUWT), such as boiling or chlorine disinfection, has long been recommended in emergencies. While there is increasing evidence that these and other PoUWT options improve household water microbiological quality and reduce diarrhoeal disease in the development context, it is unknown whether these results are generalizable to emergencies. The authors conducted a literature review and survey of implementers, and found that PoUWT was effective in small-scale, non-acute, high diarrhoeal disease-risk emergencies when training and materials were provided to recipients, adequate stocks were maintained, and chlorine dosage was appropriate. There was little documented effectiveness in acute emergencies, with untested products, or during large-scale distributions without training. Results were incorporated into the Sphere Revision, which recommends selecting culturally acceptable PoUWT options, providing adequate products and training to recipients, pre-placing PoUWT products in emergency-prone areas, and using locally available products if continued use in the post-emergency phase is desired.

Keywords: emergencies, household water treatment, implementation; point-of-use water treatment

An estimated 4 billion cases of diarrhoea each year, causing 1.8 million deaths mainly among children under five years of age, are caused by unsafe drinking water, poor sanitation, and poor hygiene (Boschi-Pinto et al., 2008). Environmental health interventions to reduce this disease burden include: improved water sources, point-of-use water treatment (PoUWT), handwashing promotion, and sanitation (Esrey et al., 1985, 1991; Fewtrell et al., 2005). Five PoUWT options – chlorination, flocculant/disinfectant powder, solar disinfection, ceramic filtration, and biosand filtration – have been shown in the development context to improve household water microbial quality and reduce diarrhoeal disease in users (Fewtrell and Colford, 2005; Clasen et al., 2007; Arnold and Colford, 2007), and another, boiling, is widely promoted. Based on this evidence, the World Health Organization (WHO) promotes PoUWT as one option to provide safe drinking water for the 884 million without access to improved water supplies and the millions more drinking microbiologically unsafe water from improved sources (WHO, 2008; UNICEF/WHO, 2008). While there is currently active debate in the water and sanitation

http://dx.doi.org/10.3362/9781780448831.002

community as to the most appropriate role for PoUWT options in development contexts that enables sustainable, consistent use over time, there remains consensus that PoUWT can improve microbiological quality of water and reduce disease in specific circumstances (Sobsey et al., 2008; Schmidt and Cairncross, 2009).

Safe drinking water is also an immediate priority in most emergencies (Sphere, 2004). When normal water supplies are interrupted or compromised following natural disasters, complex emergencies, or outbreaks, responders have often encouraged affected populations to boil or disinfect their drinking water to ensure its microbiological integrity. The Sphere Handbook provides international guidance for organizations conducting emergency response (Sphere, 2004), and recommends a minimum provision of 15 litres of water/person/day. As the emergency progresses from relief to development, the response shifts to providing higher-quality services such as long-term access to protected water supplies (Lantagne, 2009). Recently, PoUWT options verified in the development context have been recommended by numerous organizations for use in all stages of emergency response.

PoUWT, as an intervention that reduces the diarrhoeal disease burden, could potentially be an effective emergency response intervention: 1) in response to emergencies with increased risk of diarrhoeal disease, including flooding events or natural disasters that lead to displacement (Noji, 1997); 2) in some complex emergency settings when relief cannot progress to development; and 3) in response to outbreaks caused by untreated drinking water, especially cholera outbreaks, which are currently increasing in severity and quantity throughout Africa (Gaffga et al., 2007). PoUWT may also be especially effective during the initial phase of an emergency when responders cannot yet reach the affected population with longer-term solutions.

However, differences between the emergency and development contexts may affect PoUWT effectiveness, including: 1) higher crude mortality rates (Toole and Waldman, 1990) and likelihood of outbreaks due to population migration (Watson et al., 2007) in emergencies; 2) a higher level of funding affecting what water and sanitation options are selected in emergencies (de Ville de Goyet, 2000); and 3) competing priorities for staff time in emergencies (CARE, undated).

These differences raise questions about generalizability of PoUWT results from development into emergency situations. This study was conducted to explore the evidence on PoUWT in emergencies, the extent and circumstances in which emergency responders currently implement the intervention, and lessons learned to date.

Methods

Literature review

Literature on PoUWT in emergencies was identified by conducting database searches on Ovid MedLine and PubMed using the following search terms: ((('disaster*' or 'natural disaster*' or 'complex emergenc*' or 'emergenc*' or 'cholera' or 'outbreak') and ('household water treatment' or 'point of use' or 'point-of-use' or 'water treatment')). We also contacted manufacturers, UN organizations, researchers, and programme implementers (including survey respondents) to obtain grey and unpublished literature.

Survey

Data was collected from implementers of PoUWT projects in emergencies using a Word Form survey distributed via email. The survey included a mixture of attribute, belief, and knowledge questions to gain information on survey respondents and their perspective and experiences. The survey began with open-ended questions about PoUWT in emergencies generally, and continued with forced-choice questions for each individual project (each using one or more PoUWT options) implemented by the responder.

A list of 307 email addresses of individuals involved in water or emergency response from UN organizations, development and emergency-focused non-governmental organizations, research institutions, and manufacturers was created based on the literature review, email lists from the Water, Sanitation, and Hygiene in Emergencies Cluster coordinated by UNICEF, and the authors' personal contacts. The survey was emailed to this list on 29 May 2008. Recipients were encouraged to forward the survey to others able to supply information on PoUWT in emergency response. In addition, targeted emails were sent to additional identified individuals. Responses were accepted until 30 September 2008. Data collected was analysed by: 1) respondent, with answers to open-ended questions; 2) project, with answers to forced-choice questions; and 3) projects where only one PoUWT option was implemented, to compare between individual PoUWT options. The survey was approved by the LSHTM Ethics Committee.

Results

Literature review

Execution of the search strategy yielded a total of 28 journal articles, project evaluations, and manuals that met inclusion criteria of describing PoUWT interventions in emergencies (Table 2.1). By PoUWT method, this included nine (32.1 per cent) on the Procter & Gamble flocculant/disinfection product PuR, seven (25.0 per cent) on sodium hypochlorite (the CDC Safe Water System, SWS), four (14.3 per cent) on ceramic filtration, three (10.7 per cent) on boiling and safe storage promotion, three (10.7 per cent) on the 2004 Asian Tsunami specifically, one (3.6 per cent) on solar disinfection, and one (3.6 per cent) on a commercial filter. Although chlorine tablet distribution and bucket chlorination are common in emergencies (WHO, 2005), and biosand filtration is a common development intervention, no evaluations were identified using these options, although two of the PuR studies also investigated chlorine tablet distribution. Literature deemed of greater methodological quality is summarized herein categorized by PoUWT option. Effectiveness is measured by diarrhoeal disease reduction, microbiological indicator reduction, and user acceptance.

PuR

PuR is the only PoUWT option shown to effectively reduce diarrhoeal disease in an emergency in a randomized, controlled intervention trial. In this trial, conducted during the rainy season, 400 households in two Liberian refugee camps were provided with a bucket, mixing spoon, decanting cloth, funnel, safe storage container, and 21 sachets of PuR per week (Doocy and Burnham, 2006). Materials that were stolen during the course of the intervention were promptly replaced. The primary caretaker received an initial training, which included a demonstration of the correct use of PuR, distribution of pictorial instruction materials, and a requirement to demonstrate they could correctly use PuR. Weekly active diarrhoeal disease surveillance and water quality testing occurred in intervention and matched control households (provided with a safe storage container only) for 12 weeks following training. Households using PuR reported 91 per cent less diarrhoeal incidence than control households, and diarrhoea prevalence was reduced by 83 per cent compared with baseline data. A compliance rate of 95 per cent was measured, verified by weekly chlorine residual testing. The mean free chlorine residual level was 1.6 mg/L. Respondents reported appreciating the visual improvement and taste of the treated water, and the observed diarrhoeal disease reduction.

Although five other PuR evaluations collected diarrhoeal disease data, only one collected controlled data, and none reported statistical significance. Other outcome metrics used for PuR emergency projects included: 1) an increase in families collecting their PuR ration from 69 per cent to 96 per cent over the 21-week intervention period in Uganda (SP, 2006); 2) 78 per cent of interviewed households correctly stating how to use PuR and 10 per cent having chlorine residual in household water in Haiti after flooding (Colindres et al., 2007); and 3) 95 per cent of interviewed families having chlorine residual in household water during seasonal flooding in Vietnam (Handzel and Bamrah, 2006; UNICEF, 2007).

Two of the richest PuR evaluations were conducted in Bangladesh after flooding events. In the first project evaluated, 20 PuR sachets and 20 Aquatabs were included in the relief packages for 4,800 families in 67 flood-affected villages in Bangladesh from September 2006 to February 2007 (Hoque and Khanam, undated). All recipients received group demonstration at distribution, and a subset of recipients received follow-up community level trainings conducted by project motivators. To assess the project, 239 families were visited to obtain 200 (83.7 per cent) families that were using one of the products at the unannounced household visit. Of the 200 families surveyed, 200 (100 per cent) had received PuR and 176 (88.0 per cent) had received Aquatabs. Three-quarters (150) were using PuR that day, with 50 (25 per cent)

POINT-OF-USE WATER TREATMENT IN EMERGENCY RESPONSE 17

Table 2.1 Journal articles, programme evaluations, and manuals identified describing PoUWT interventions in emergencies

PoUWT option	Emergency type	Country	Methods	Outcome metrics	Source
PuR	Refugee camp	Liberia	RCT, WQ testing	Diarrhoea, FRC	(Doocy and Burnham, 2006)
PuR	Refugee camp	Uganda	Project evaluation	Families collecting PuR	(SP, 2006)
PuR	Flooding	Haiti	Survey	Knowledge, FRC	(CARE, undated, Colindres et al., 2007)
PuR	Feeding programme	Ethiopia	Survey, WQ testing	FRC	(CARE, undated)
PuR	Complex	DRC	Survey	Knowledge	(IMC, 2008)
PuR/chlorine tablets	Flooding	Bangladesh	Survey, WQ testing	FRC, uptake, diarrhoea	(Hoque and Khanam, undated)
PuR/chlorine tablets	Flooding	Bangladesh	Survey, WQ testing	FRC, uptake, diarrhoea	(Johnston, 2008)
PuR	Seasonal flooding	Vietnam	Survey, WQ testing	FRC, uptake	(Handzel and Bamrah, 2006; UNICEF, 2007)
PuR	–	–	Manual	–	(Aquaya, 2005)
Sodium hypochlorite	Flooding/cholera	Madagascar	Survey, WQ testing	FRC, uptake	(Dunston et al., 2001)
Sodium hypochlorite	Cholera	Madagascar	Case-control	Cholera risk	(Reller et al., 2001)
Sodium hypochlorite	Flooding	Madagascar	Survey, WQ testing	FRC, uptake	(Mong et al., 2001)
Sodium hypochlorite/ boiling	Tsunami	Indonesia	Survey, WQ testing	FRC, *E. coli*, uptake	(Gupta et al., 2007)
Sodium hypochlorite	Complex	Haiti	Survey, WQ testing	Diarrhoea, FRC	(Brin, 2003)
Sodium hypochlorite	Complex	Haiti	Survey, WQ testing	FRC, uptake	(Ritter, 2007)

(continued)

18   WATER, SANITATION AND HYGIENE IN HUMANITARIAN CONTEXTS

Table 2.1 Journal articles, programme evaluations, and manuals identified describing PoUWT interventions in emergencies (continued)

PoUWT option	Emergency type	Country	Methods	Outcome metrics	Source
Sodium hypochlorite	–	–	Manual	–	(CDC, 2008)
Ceramic filtration	Tsunami	Sri Lanka	Survey	Uptake, use	(Palmer, 2005)
Ceramic filtration	Flooding	Dominican Rep.	RCT Survey, WQ testing	Faecal coliform Uptake, correct use	(Clasen and Boisson, 2006)
Ceramic filtration	Flooding	Haiti	Survey	Uptake, WTP	(Caens, 2005)
Ceramic filtration	–	Multiple	Filter factory evaluation	Best practices	(Lantagne, 2006)
Safe storage	Refugee camp	Sudan	Clinic record review	Diarrhoea	(Walden et al., 2005)
Safe storage/mother solution	Refugee camp	Malawi	RCT, WQ testing	Diarrhoea, faecal coliform	(Roberts et al., 2001)
Boiling	Flooding	USA	Survey	Knowledge	(Ram et al., 2007)
SODIS	Cholera	Kenya	Sub-group of RCT	Diarrhoea	(Conroy et al., 2001)
Multiple interventions	Tsunami	India, Sri Lanka, Indonesia	Interviews, site visit	Evaluation	(Clasen and Smith, 2005)
Multiple interventions	Tsunami	Indonesia	WQ testing	WQ testing	(Gupta and Quick, 2006)
Multiple interventions	–	–	Manual	–	(WHO, 2005)
Nerox filter	IDP camp	Pakistan	Survey	Uptake	(Zehri and Ensink, 2008)

Note: FRC (free residual chlorine), WQ (water quality), RCT (randomized, controlled trial), WTP (willingness to pay) using Aquatabs. Water quality testing showed that no treated water sample had detectible faecal coliform, and all samples had free chlorine residual. The second evaluation was conducted after Cyclone Sidr in 2007 (Johnston, 2008). At least 5 million Aquatabs were widely distributed without specific training for recipients, and 120,000 PuR sachets were distributed with training. No faecal coliforms were detected in water treated with Aquatabs or PuR, and a greater number of households were using and preferred PuR to Aquatabs. A total of 100 per cent of households had PuR in the house, with 72 per cent having treated water at the time of the unannounced visit. A smaller percentage, 65 per cent of households, had Aquatabs in the house, with 10 per cent having treated water at the time of the unannounced visit.

All PuR in emergency project evaluations, except after flooding in Haiti, occurred in stable emergencies where community health workers could access families reliably over time. In Uganda, Ethiopia, and Vietnam, projects distributed one sachet/day/family, which was determined sufficient for most families' drinking water needs. In Liberia, Uganda, Ethiopia, Bangladesh, and DRC, buckets or buckets with stirring rods and cloth were distributed along with sachets. In Vietnam, households had the materials needed to use PuR because they were accustomed to using alum for flocculation.

Group demonstrations and weekly follow-up generated high uptake in Liberia, Bangladesh, and Vietnam, with 95.4 per cent, 62.8–72 per cent, and 95 per cent, respectively, of respondents having chlorine residual in household water. In Bangladesh, uptake of PuR was higher in households receiving centralized training and community follow-up (89 per cent) than in communities receiving only centralized training (54 per cent). In Haiti, where only community trainings were conducted, 10 per cent of recipients had chlorine residual in household water. Local registration was noted necessary for project implementation in Haiti and Vietnam.

In Liberia, respondents reported appreciating the taste, in Haiti 97 per cent of people reported PuR-treated water tasted better than non-treated water, and in Ethiopia taste was acceptable. In contrast, taste was a barrier in Bangladesh, and in Vietnam it was postulated people disliked the taste so intensely they boiled water after PuR treatment.

PuR willingness to pay ranged from: 1) an average 2.7 US cents (USC) in Haiti; 2) 44.5 per cent of respondents stating 0.4 USC in Bangladesh; and 3) 80 per cent of respondents in Vietnam stating 1.3–3.2 USC.

Chlorine tablets

The only chlorine tablet research identified was conducted concurrently with the Bangladesh PuR studies referenced above (Handzel and Bamrah, 2006; UNICEF, 2007; Hoque and Khanam, undated). In the two studies, 88 per cent and 65 per cent of PuR study households also received Aquatabs, and 25 per cent and 10 per cent, respectively, were using Aquatabs at the household visit. Aquatabs training was not provided, although PuR training was. All Aquatabs-treated household water had adequate chlorine residual and no faecal coliforms. Respondents preferred PuR (p<0.001), but were willing to use Aquatabs; and 30.5 per cent were willing to pay 0.4 US¢ per tablet.

Sodium hypochlorite

All hypochlorite research identified in emergencies used in-country produced SWS development products, which have been implemented in response to natural disasters, complex emergencies, and outbreaks.

Five months after receiving a cyclone relief kit containing sodium hypochlorite and foldable jerry cans, 25 per cent of recipients in Madagascar had chlorine residual in household water (Mong et al., 2001). Recipients were willing to pay US$0.38 for additional hypochlorite bottles. In addition, confirmed chlorine residual presence was 14 per cent, 14.7 per cent, and 2.64 per cent five months after the tsunami in three villages receiving free product during the emergency (Gupta et al., 2007). Factors associated with decreased risk of *E. coli* contamination in household water included: 1) reported sodium hypochlorite use; 2) chlorine residual presence; 3) observed use of washing hands with soap; and 4) latrine use. During the 2008 cyclone, PSI/Myanmar distributed enough locally made sodium hypochlorite to treat over 200 million litres of water; however, the efficacy of the intervention is unknown as no evaluation was conducted.

In the complex emergency of northern Haiti, sodium hypochlorite is locally produced. Families purchase hypochlorite for $0.10/month in refillable bottles, and technicians paid from programme income produce and sell the hypochlorite, train new users, and conduct household visits with existing users. After a 2003 evaluation documented significant reductions in microbiological contamination in users' household water (Brin, 2003), the project expanded, and in 2007, 67 per cent of programme households had chlorine residual in household water (Ritter, 2007). During disasters, project staff work with local churches and resellers to distribute tickets for free solution to affected families (Gallo, 2008).

During cholera outbreaks in Madagascar, documented usage (measured by chlorine residual in household water) was 11.2–19.7 per cent of households receiving community-based mobilization (Dunston et al., 2001). During one particular 2001 outbreak, sodium hypochlorite use (odds ratio = 0.1, 95%CI = 0.0–1.2) and boiling (odds ratio = 0.4, CI = 0.1–1.1) were associated with statistically insignificant reductions (p = 0.11 and 0.09, respectively, and attributed to small sample size) in cholera risk (Reller et al., 2001).

Ceramic filters

Evaluations of ceramic filter distributions in emergencies have been conducted in three locations. The first, in Sri Lanka after the 2004 tsunami (Palmer, 2005), found that the factors associated with use included: having used wells for drinking water before the tsunami, future planned well use, practising any type of water treatment, a greater length of time between the tsunami and filter distribution, higher quality of shelter, more programmatic support, and distribution of pot (instead of candle) filters. Barriers to use were insufficient filter training and lack of living space.

Ceramic candle filters were also distributed to families affected by flooding in the Dominican Republic in 2003 (Clasen and Boisson, 2006). Community mobilizers identified and trained recipient families, who were advised the candles were effective for six months. Local businesses sold replacement filters for ~$4.50. In a randomized, controlled trial among 80 households, faecal coliform was found to be consistently lower among intervention than control households ($p<0.0001$). A cross-sectional study 16 months after filter distribution found 102 (88.7 per cent) recipient households still had their filters, 68 (66.7 per cent) were using them, 56 (48.7 per cent) filters were operating properly, and 30 (29.4 per cent) families had treated water free of faecal coliforms. Thirty-three (58.9 per cent) of the 56 households with an operating filter had replaced the filter.

In Haiti, ceramic filter systems were distributed after flooding in 2003 (Caens, 2005). Although users self-reported liking the filter and health benefits, willingness to pay for the filter was less than filter replacement costs, and area kiosks were not willing to stock the filter.

Standard emergency response interventions

Three studies were identified investigating the standard and more traditional PoUWT emergency response interventions: boiling, safe storage promotion, and mother solution (on-site-produced sodium hypochlorite). In the previously referenced study after the tsunami, narrow-mouthed water storage container use, reported boiling, adequate boiling, and adequate boiling with water storage were not associated with decreased risk of *E. coli* in stored water (Gupta et al., 2007).

During an outbreak of shigellosis in a refugee camp in Sudan (Walden et al., 2005), a campaign involving house-to-house visits to clean their safe storage containers and distribute information was conducted. Although gathering statistically rigorous data was not possible, clinic health records showed a reduction of watery and bloody diarrhoea in the weeks following the cleaning project.

In a Malawian refugee camp, intervention households were provided with 1–3 improved 20-litre buckets with a lid and spout (Roberts et al., 2001). Mean faecal coliform counts were 53.3 per cent lower in improved buckets compared with normal buckets, and children in improved bucket households had a statistically insignificant 31.1 per cent reduction of diarrhoeal disease ($p=0.06$). Mother solution distributed by a health committee member in the camp was 27 per cent and 8 per cent of the required concentration in two tests.

Emerging technologies

Emerging PoUWT technologies – such as one microfilter gravity system that had been tested for microbiological efficacy, but undergone little field testing – have been implemented in emergencies (Zehri and Ensink, 2008). In Pakistan internally displaced camps, nine months after filter distribution, 21 (10 per cent) householders reported they used the filter every day, and on visual inspection, 12 (5.7 per cent) of the filters were in working condition. Users reported that water takes too long to filter (78 per cent), cleaning is difficult (23 per cent), the filter needs to be cleaned too often (24 per cent), and water becomes too hot (82 per cent).

Specific case: 2005 tsunami

The most thorough evaluation of PoUWT in a single emergency commenced eight weeks after the 2004 tsunami in India, Sri Lanka, and Indonesia (Clasen and Smith, 2005). Despite wide availability of products, PoUWT 'did not play a significant role in the initial phases of the tsunami response with the possible exception of boiling'. Boiling was widely promoted because it 'was well-known and widely accepted, it did not require programmatic support for its promotion, thus allowing them [NGOs] to focus on providing basic water and sanitation needs'.

Millions of PuR sachets, chlorine tablets, and sodium hypochlorite bottles were not used in the immediate aftermath of the tsunami because: 1) water quantity was considered more important than water quality; 2) PoUWT was unnecessary because water was supplied from tanker trucks; 3) the scale of the emergency precluded human and other resource availability for PoUWT programmatic support; and 4) implementers were concerned about sending mixed messages diluting boiling promotion effectiveness and about promoting unsustainable PoUWT options.

In contrast to PoUWT options, water distribution options, such as water tankering, were widely used. In Aceh after the tsunami, 33 (44 per cent) tanker truck water samples had <0.1 mg/L chlorine residual, and 9 (17 per cent) tested positive for *E. coli* (Gupta and Quick, 2006). Factors leading to contamination included: 1) long wait times at filling stations causing drivers to fill trucks from untreated sources; 2) underchlorinated filling station water; and 3) sediment from untreated sources in tanker trucks exerting chlorine demand.

Survey results

Fifty-four respondents returned the email survey, with a response rate of 4.2 per cent (13) from the initial email, 1.9 per cent (6) from traceable email forwards, and 100 per cent (3) from targeted emails. It is unknown how 32 (59.3 per cent) respondents obtained the survey. Fourteen (26 per cent) responses were excluded from analysis because: they did not use PoUWT in an emergency (3); survey form was incomplete (1); and there were duplicate survey responses from resellers of one PoUWT option (11). The 40 remaining respondents included: 15 (37.5 per cent) from international development organizations; 17 (42.5 per cent) from international emergency organizations; 5 (12.8 per cent) researchers; 2 (5.1 per cent) manufacturers; and 1 (2.6 per cent) individual. Respondents described projects using 19 PoUWT options (Figure 2.1). The nine other PoUWT options in the figure included: mission filter, alum, mother solution, locally made flocculant/disinfectant (2), chulli filter, UV, and SteriPen (2).

The 40 respondents described 77 projects using one or more PoUWT options (average 1.93 projects/respondent, range 1–8). Two projects were duplicates, and the survey response from the implementer was included in subsequent analysis.

The 75 remaining projects occurred in 25 countries, encompassing a variety of emergencies (Table 2.2). Fifty-one (68 per cent) projects began in the acute emergency stage, 6 (8 per cent) in late emergency, and 5 (6.7 per cent) post-emergency. The average number of weeks to respond to the emergency with PoUWT was 3.7 (range 0–36). The majority (68 per cent) of PoUWT projects were implemented in rural areas. The remaining were in urban areas (21.3 per cent) or mixed urban/rural (10.7 per cent) locations. Recipients lived primarily in communities (58.7 per cent), followed by internally displaced (28.0 per cent), refugee (6.7 per cent), and mixed (6.7 per cent) settings.

Projects began between 1999 and 2008. The 66 projects started between 1999–2007 fit an exponential growth curve ($R^2=0.92$).

Technical assistance was obtained locally within the respondents' organizations in 39 (50.6 per cent) projects, locally outside the respondents' organization in 22 (28.6 per cent) projects, within the respondents' organization internationally in 23 (29.9 per cent) projects, and outside their organization internationally in 4 (5.2 per cent) projects. One project implementing mother solution indicated technical assistance was needed, but not available. Respondents reported that project assessments were completed for 68 (90.7 per cent) projects.

Survey respondents reported an average of 2.16 water sources (range 1–3) used per project. Seventy (43.3 per cent) of the 162 total sources listed were

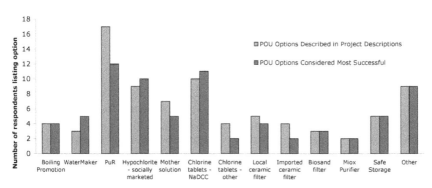

Figure 2.1 Which PoUWT options were considered most successful?

Table 2.2 Projects reported in the survey by emergency type and continent

	Africa	Americas	Asia	Total
Natural disaster: cyclone/ waterlogging	1	1	10	12 (16%)
Natural disaster: food	10	6	11	27 (36%)
Natural disaster: tsunami			9	9 (12%)
Natural disaster: earthquake		3	4	7 (9.3%)
Natural disaster: food and Outbreak: cholera	2			2 (2.7%)
Outbreak: cholera	11			11 (14.7%)
Outbreak: Ebola, hepatitis E, typhoid	3			3 (4%)
Complex emergency	4			4 (5.3%)
Total	31 (41.3%)	10 (13.3%)	35 (45.3%)	75

'improved' (such as infrastructure, protected well, protected spring). The remaining 92 sources (56.7 per cent) were unimproved (surface water, open well, unprotected spring). Data from the 56 projects using only one PoUWT option were analysed separately. Fifty-four single-option projects were stratified into four PoUWT option categories: filters, flocculant/disinfectant, sodium hypochlorite, and chlorine tablets. One boiling and one alum project were not categorized. Flocculant/disinfectants were targeted more often (68.2 per cent) to unprotected water sources, and chlorine tablets were targeted more often (72.2 per cent) to areas with protected water sources, although this result was not statistically significant. Filters and sodium hypochlorite were targeted slightly less, 45.8 per cent and 44.4 per cent of projects, respectively, to protected sources.

Data collected from the following questions was considered too unreliable to report: units of PoUWT product distributed, target population size, cost of product to the organization, time to receive the products, and whether products were available locally or imported.

The particular PoUWT option(s) used were selected for 184 reasons (Figure 2.2). An average of 2.45 reasons were listed per project (range 0–5). Availability of product was the most frequent reason for use, mentioned in 64 per cent of projects. Local water quality or user acceptability accounted for few reasons for use.

When stratified by single-option projects, flocculant/disinfectants were selected more often because of product availability, appropriateness for water quality, or donation. Product sustainability was mentioned as a reason for selection of locally manufactured or longer-lasting products, such as sodium hypochlorite and filters. Chlorine tablets were the only option where 'familiarity to users' was considered. These data were not statistically significant owing to small sample size.

'Product' responses were considered the easiest factors in implementation, while 'user' responses and product distribution were considered the most difficult factors (Figure 2.3). Users were trained using group demonstrations in 62 (80.5 per cent), written materials in 28 (36.4 per cent), and one-on-one training in 20 (26.0 per cent) projects. Focus group demonstrations were completed in nine (11.7 per cent), and no training was conducted in six (7.8 per cent) projects.

When stratified by single-option projects, user acceptability was noted as an easy factor in implementation in filter projects, chorine tablets were noted most often as easy to distribute, and difficulties with user acceptability were noted the most for chlorine tablets. Product distribution and user training was noted as a difficult issue for filter projects. These data were not statistically significant owing to small sample size.

The main user concerns expressed related to aesthetics, preference for piped water, and managing the use of the product (Table 2.3). Other concerns included (each mentioned once): lower efficacy in this product than another used before, never seen product before, boiling familiar and practical while this product is

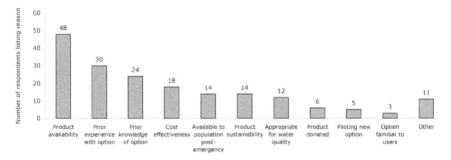

Figure 2.2 Reasons given for selecting PoUWT option

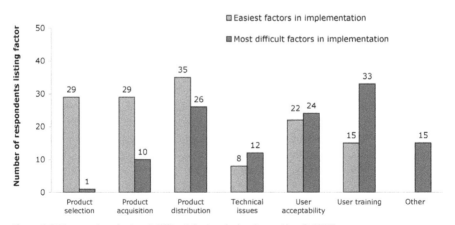

Figure 2.3 The most easiest and difficult factors in implementing PoUWT

Table 2.3 Survey data on concerns and positive aspects of PoUWT products expressed by users, reported by implementers

Concerns about products expressed by users (reported by respondent)		Positive aspects of products expressed by users (reported by respondent)	
Concern	Number and % of 75 projects	Positive aspect	Number and % of 75 projects
Aesthetics (taste, colour, odour)	34 (44.2%)	Providing safe water	42 (54.5%)
Preference for piped water	9 (11.7%)	Health benefit	38 (49.4%)
Too much time to use	8 (10.4%)	Ease of use	29 (37.7%)
Cleaning/maintaining product	7 (9.1%)	Aesthetic benefit	10 (13.0%)
Difficult to use	4 (5.2%)	Cost	1 (1.3%)
None	5 (6.5%)		
Other	11 (14.3%)		

new, not enough water treated, price too high to purchase post-emergency, not enough water available, product did not have a faucet, product might be harmful, product was not sufficiently available, and there was religious objection to the product. The majority of positive user responses expressed about PoUWT products, as reported by respondents, were health-related.

Discussion

Overall, product options dominate how PoUWT research in emergencies has been conducted. One-third of the research identified in the literature review was sponsored or conducted by one private company, Procter & Gamble, on the PuR product. Only 4 of the 28 (14.3 per cent) reports identified for the literature review reported on multiple-PoUWT option reports. Only 19 (25.3 per cent) of 75 projects described in the survey used multiple PoUWT options, and the majority of the reasons respondents picked PoUWT options were product related; 64 per cent of projects reported 'product availability' as the reason for use. This focus on showing how a specific PoUWT option is effective in specific emergencies obscures the more important research questions of which PoUWT options are most effective at microbiological and disease reduction, most appropriate, cost effective, usable by the target population, and sustainable across different stages and types of emergency. In the following sections, a cross-option comparison of data addresses these questions. Further research on PoUWT should focus less on individual products and more on holistic programming.

Literature review

There is some evidence that PoUWT is effective in non-acute emergency settings. PuR use has been shown to reduce diarrhoeal disease in one refugee camp and improve microbiological quality of household water in cyclones. Sodium hypochlorite use improved microbiological quality of water after the tsunami and during a complex emergency. Ceramic filters have been shown to improve microbiological quality of water during and after flooding. In addition, survey respondents' consider the majority of PoUWT options they have used to be successful, suggesting high acceptability of PoUWT among those promoting and distributing them. Non-significant diarrhoeal disease results in sodium hypochlorite response to cholera and a refugee camp safe storage project could be attributed to small sample size, although that is unknown.

Health impact and microbiological reduction are gold standards for measuring PoUWT impact; however, these metrics can be difficult to assess in emergencies. Some projects described herein were able to gather valuable impact metrics, such as chlorine residual in household water and quantitative information on use and acceptance. Other metrics collected, such as non-controlled self-reported diarrhoeal disease data or knowledge of method to reduce diarrhoea, might be less valuable. Appropriate metrics to assess PoUWT impact, considering what is realistic to collect and analyse in emergencies, rather than the perceived need to obtain health outcomes, should be utilized.

Training is key for PoUWT uptake in, and continued use after, emergencies. High usage of PuR in emergencies was associated with a training session and additional follow-up education. Sodium hypochlorite use in emergencies was seen in 3–20 per cent of household waters, although higher long-term uptake levels (76.7 per cent in Haiti) were documented when families had follow-up training. A correct usage of 26.3 per cent in ceramic filter users was documented with only one initial training, indicating less follow-up may be needed for durable PoUWT options. Lack of microbiological improvement in boiled water in Indonesia indicates that not all users are boiling correctly, and additional training is needed.

Product costs – not including transportation, distribution, or marketing – of PuR (treats 10 litres), Aquatabs (20 litres), and sodium hypochlorite bottles (1,000 litres) are $0.035, $0.015, and $0.33, respectively. Willingness to pay estimates (for PuR, Aquatabs, ceramic filter replacement parts) were less than product cost except for sodium hypochlorite bottles. Although cost may not factor significantly in emergency response programmes, cost-recovery is critical if continued access to PoUWT in the post-emergency stage is desired.

Each PoUWT option has benefits and drawbacks, and thus, situations where they are most appropriately implemented. In emergencies, ceramic filters appear to be a more appropriate intervention after the acute emergency has passed, when householders are moving from transitional to permanent situations. Locally made or locally available products with low cost, such as the SWS or chlorine tablets, may be more appropriate for a relief-to-development model where continued access to the products is desired. PuR may be most appropriate in populations using highly turbid water, where community follow-up training can be conducted during the emergency. Boiling may be particularly appropriate among populations familiar with it already, or entrapped populations when they have the materials to practise the method. Safe storage is an important complement to any PoUWT method, especially those that do not provide for residual protection against re-contamination. Using new products in an emergency is not recommended unless user acceptability is assessed before distribution.

Chlorine dosage

The commercially available chlorine-based PoUWT options – PuR, chlorine tablets, and sodium hypochlorite – all use a fixed chlorine dosage. PuR uses 2.0 mg/L, which adequately maintained chlorine residual in 30 representative water sources of turbidity 0.3–1,724 NTU in western Kenya (Crump et al., 2004). The dosage of chlorine tablets is, generally, 2.0 mg/L for clear water (1 tab) and 4.0 mg/L for turbid water (2 tabs). The dosage for SWS products is 1.875 mg/L for clear water (1 cap) and 3.75 mg/L for turbid water (2 caps), which maintained adequate chlorine residual levels (>0.2 mg/L and <2.0 mg/L for 24 hours after treatment) in 86.6 per cent of 82 clear and 91.7 per cent of 12 turbid water samples tested from representative sources in 13 developing countries (Lantagne, 2008). Treating water >100 NTU directly with sodium hypochlorite was not recommended. Although these fixed dosages lead to chlorine residuals that exceed the recommended WHO chlorine residual for infrastructure treated water at the point of delivery (0.2–0.5 mg/L) (WHO, 2004), these dosage regimes: 1) are below the maximum guideline value of 5.0 mg/L; 2) maintain chlorine residual during 24 hours of storage in the home; and 3) have been specifically approved as 'consistent with the Third Edition of the [WHO] Guidelines [for drinking-water quality]' for household water treatment purposes, where storage of water at the household level causes degradation of chlorine residual over time (Jamie Bartram, World Health Organization, Geneva, personal communication with Eric Mintz, CDC, Atlanta, 2005).

In contrast, emergency organizations generally test each source empirically using a stock solution to determine what dosage leads to chlorine residual of 0.4–0.5 mg/L 30 minutes after treatment (WHO, 2005), or use special chlorine tablets dosing at 5 mg/L (Paul Edmondson, Medentech, Ltd, Ireland, personal communication with D. Lantagne, 2008). Although 5 mg/L does not exceed the WHO guideline value for chlorine residual in drinking water, it does exceed the taste acceptability threshold (WHO, 2004, Lantagne, 2008).

The lack of user acceptability of high chlorine dosages significantly affects chlorination projects in emergencies, and appropriate dosage regimes should be developed. Dosing at 5 mg/L will likely exceed the taste acceptability threshold, and 0.5 mg/L dosage will likely not maintain sufficient residual during household storage of water.

Survey

The survey was widely distributed to individuals involved with PoUWT in development and emergency contexts, and survey respondents represented a diverse group of implementers in the emergency, development, research, and manufacturing sectors, using a large variety of PoUWT options. Implementers consider the majority of the options they have used in emergencies to be 'most successful' according to their own personal definition of success.

The 75 projects described by the 40 respondents represented a diverse geographic coverage across Africa, Asia, and the Americas. Sixty-four (85.3 per cent) projects were implemented in emergencies identified as having high diarrhoeal disease risk from the literature review (such as flooding events and outbreaks). The majority of the projects (68 per cent) began in the acute emergency stage, when the risk of outbreak is highest. Projects generally targeted persons at higher risk of disease and with less access to improved water supplies, such as those living in rural areas, communities, and the internally displaced. Overall, the projects targeted areas with unimproved water supplies (56.7 per cent of supplies), and the specific PoUWT option used in single-option projects was appropriate for the local water sources.

Technical assistance on PoUWT implementation in emergency response was primarily found locally or from within the respondents' organizations. This result highlights that technical assistance should be available locally and specifically targeted for each implementing organization. Although 89.3 per cent of respondents noted that they had assessed their project in some manner, few of these assessments were independent or made available for our review. Thus, the implementers' perception of success cannot be matched with quantitative data showing project feasibility, and knowledge gained from these evaluations cannot be collated and shared as lessons learned.

There is evidence that PoUWT projects in emergencies are growing at an exponential rate, but this may be the result of systematic or reporting bias. Implementers found it difficult to respond to many logistical questions, and thus an amount of water treated in respondents' projects could not be calculated. The scope of PoUWT product distribution in emergencies is not small, as distributors and manufacturers reported supplying enough sodium hypochlorite, chlorine tablets, and PuR sachets to treat 3.3 billion, 1.65 billion, and 171 million litres of water, respectively, in response to emergencies in 2007 alone (Clasen, 2008). It is unknown how much of these products were used at the household level, however.

Product reasons (such as availability and knowledge) dominate the PoUWT option selection process as opposed to user reasons, and product factors were considered the easiest factors in implementing PoUWT. Concurrently, user acceptance and user training were identified as the most difficult factors in implementation, and should be considered more fully in project planning. The easiest and most difficult factors in implementation varied between PoUWT options, indicating that implementation strategies should be specialized for each PoUWT option.

Given that interventions in developing countries are often promoted for health reasons, but users change behaviour for other motivations (Scott et al., 2007), the utility of the respondents' reporting health reasons as the main user positive for PoUWT is unclear.

The main limitations of the survey were: 1) non-response and voluntary response bias potentially preventing implementers with failed PoUWT projects from answering the survey; 2) conclusions drawn by implementers are largely subjective, and are, in most cases, not supported by a rigorous and independent assessment; and 3) not enough survey responses were received to conduct stratified statistical analyses.

Based on the investigations reported herein, the authors worked in conjunction with the Sphere project to develop guidelines for organizations interested in implementing PoUWT programmes for inclusion in the new Sphere revision. The revision will state: 1) that PoUWT can be used as an option when centralized treatment is not possible; 2) the options that have been shown to reduce diarrhoea and improve microbiological water quality; 3) that the most appropriate PoUWT option for any given context depends on existing water and sanitation conditions, water quality, cultural acceptability, implementation feasibility, availability of option, and local conditions; 4) that successful emergency household level water treatment implementations should include the selection of culturally acceptable options, provision of adequate material product and appropriate training to the beneficiary recipients; 5) that introducing an untested water treatment option in an emergency should be avoided; 6) that in areas with anticipated risk, pre-placement of PoUWT products should be considered to facilitate a quick response; and 7) the use of locally available products should be prioritized if continued use in the post-emergency phase is desired. A decision tree for PoUWT products was developed and vetted by a committee of experts, and will also be included.

Additional evidence on the following topics is needed: 1) project monitoring and evaluation; 2) efficacy of unproven 'standard interventions'; 3) lessons learned from projects with multiple PoUWT interventions; 4) PoUWT effectiveness in acute emergencies; 5) relative appropriateness of different PoUWT options in emergencies and with different types of training; and 6) PoUWT effectiveness compared with other water and sanitation interventions. Research is also needed to investigate survey respondents' perceptions that: 1) pre-emergency knowledge of a PoUWT option (either via a long-term development project or repeated exposure to the product during emergencies) increases user acceptability and adoption, and decreases the training requirement; and 2) PoUWT use in emergencies encourages long-term water treatment in the household. Lastly, the focus herein has been exclusively on PoUWT in emergencies, and the concurrent potential for water quality improvements and diarrhoeal disease reduction. Further research is indicated to develop guidelines for implementing organizations on how to: 1) include PoUWT as part of the overall strategy in emergency response; and 2) decide whether to use PoUWT at a particular time within a particular emergency.

Conclusions

In development settings, PoUWT options have been shown to improve the microbiological quality of household water and reduce diarrhoeal disease in users. There is comparatively little rigorous evidence of PoUWT in emergency settings. However, from the rigorous evidence and user surveys, it is known that: 1) PoUWT can be an effective water intervention in some (non-acute) emergencies; 2) current PoUWT projects correctly target emergencies with high diarrhoeal disease risk; 3) considering user preference in PoUWT option selection facilitates implementation; 4) training is crucial to uptake of PoUWT in emergencies; 5) adequate product stocks are necessary for emergency response; 6) difficulties in obtaining local registration hinder projects; 7) users should have all the materials necessary to use the PoUWT options; and 8) chlorine dosage should be considered in light of user acceptability concerns.

In addition, it is known that: 1) there is less documented success of PoUWT in acute emergencies; 2) introducing an untested PoUWT product in an emergency may not be effective; 3) some PoUWT options may be more appropriate in particular emergencies than others; 4) PoUWT should always be one strategy of many to ensure safe water access in emergencies; and 5) the relevance of sustainable, long-term access to the products should be considered in project planning.

About the authors

Daniele Lantagne (daniele.lantagne@tufts.edu) is an environmental engineer who has worked in over 40 countries providing technical assistance on household water treatment. At the time of writing she had completed this work as a PhD candidate and research assistant at the London School of Hygiene and Tropical Medicine (LSHTM), working with her advisor **Dr Thomas Clasen** under a contract from CDC and USAID. She is now Assistant Professor, Department of Civil and Environmental Engineering at Tufts University. **Thomas Clasen** was a Senior Lecturer in Water, Sanitation and Health at the LSHTM, and is now Professor of Environmental Health at Emory University and is the Rose Salamone Gangarosa Chair of Sanitation and Safe Water.

The authors would like to thank **Tom Handzel** and **Ian Moise** for technical support and advice, and the survey respondents who made this paper possible. This work was supported by the United States Agency for International Development and the Centers for Disease Control and Prevention.

References

Aquaya (2005) *Standard Operating Procedure for the Deployment of Procter & Gamble's PUR Purifier of Water in Emergency Response Settings*, Aquaya Institute, San Francisco, CA.

Arnold, B.F. and Colford, J.M. Jr (2007) 'Treating water with chlorine at point-of-use to improve water quality and reduce child diarrhea in developing countries: A systematic review and meta-analysis', *American Journal of Tropical Medicine and Hygiene* 76: 354–64.

Boschi-Pinto, C., Velebit, L. and Shibuya, K. (2008) 'Estimating child mortality due to diarrhoea in developing countries', *Bulletin of the World Health Organization* 86: 710–17.

Brin, G. (2003) *Evaluation of the Safe Water System in Jolivert Haiti by Bacteriological Testing and Public Health Survey,* Department of Civil and Environmental Engineering, Massachusetts Institute of Technology, Cambridge, MA.

Caens, C. (2005) *An Evaluation of the User Acceptability of Oxfam's Household Ceramic Filter,* Cranfield University, Silsoe, UK.

CARE (Undated) *Global Development Alliance, Safe Drinking Water Alliance, Report of Findings: Draft Outline,* CARE, Atlanta, GA.

CDC (2008) *Safe Water for the Community: A Guide for Establishing a Community-based Safe Water System Program,* Centers for Disease Control and Prevention, Atlanta, GA.

Clasen, T. (2008) *Scaling Up Household Water Treatment: Looking Back, Seeing Forward,* Public Health and the Environment, World Health Organization, Geneva.

Clasen, T. and Boisson, S. (2006) 'Household-based ceramic water filters for the treatment of drinking water in disaster response: An assessment of a pilot programme in the Dominican Republic', *Water Practice & Technology* 1: 2 doi:10.2166/WPT.2006031.

Clasen, T. and Smith, L. (2005) *The Drinking Water Response to the Indian Ocean Tsunami, including the Role of Household Water Treatment,* World Health Organization, Geneva.

Clasen, T., Schmidt, W.P., Rabie, T., Roberts, I. and Cairncross, S. (2007) 'Interventions to improve water quality for preventing diarrhoea: Systematic review and meta-analysis', *BMJ* 334: 782.

Colindres, R.E., Jain, S., Bowen, A., Mintz, E. and Domond, P. (2007) 'After the flood: An evaluation of in-home drinking water treatment with combined flocculent-disinfectant following Tropical Storm Jeanne – Gonaives, Haiti, 2004', *Journal of Water and Health* 5: 367–74.

Conroy, R.M., Meegan, M.E., Joyce, T., McGuigan, K. and Barnes, J. (2001) 'Solar disinfection of drinking water protects against cholera in children under 6 years of age', *Archives of Disease in Childhood* 85: 293–95.

Crump, J.A., Okoth, G.O., Slutsker, L., Ogaja, D.O., Keswick, B.H. and Luby, S.P. (2004) 'Effect of point-of-use disinfection, flocculation and combined flocculation-disinfection on drinking water quality in western Kenya', *Journal of Applied Microbiology* 97: 225–31.

De Ville De Goyet, C. (2000) 'Stop propagating disaster myths', *Lancet* 356: 762–64.

Doocy, S. and Burnham, G. (2006) 'Point-of-use water treatment and diarrhoea reduction in the emergency context: An effectiveness trial in Liberia', *Tropical Medicine & International Health* 11: 1542–52.

Dunston, C., McAfee, D., Kaiser, R., Rakotoarison, D., Rambeloson, L., Hoang, A.T. and Quick, R.E. (2001) 'Collaboration, cholera, and cyclones: A project to improve point-of-use water quality in Madagascar', *American Journal of Public Health* 91: 1574–76.

Esrey, S.A., Feachem, R.G. and Hughes, J.M. (1985) 'Interventions for the control of diarrhoeal diseases among young children: improving water supplies and excreta disposal facilities', *Bulletin of the World Health Organization* 63: 757–72.

Esrey, S.A., Potash, J.B., Roberts, L. and Shiff, C. (1991) 'Effects of improved water supply and sanitation on ascariasis, diarrhoea, dracunculiasis, hookworm infection, schistosomiasis, and trachoma', *Bulletin of the World Health Organization* 69: 609–21.

Fewtrell, L. and Colford, J.M. Jr (2005) 'Water, sanitation and hygiene in developing countries: Interventions and diarrhoea – a review', *Water Science and Technology* 52: 133–42.
Fewtrell, L., Kaufmann, R.B., Kay, D., Enanoria, W., Haller, L. and Colford, J.M. Jr (2005) 'Water, sanitation, and hygiene interventions to reduce diarrhoea in less developed countries: A systematic review and meta-analysis', *Lancet Infectious Diseases* 5: 42–52.
Gaffga, N.H., Tauxe, R.V. and Mintz, E.D. (2007) 'Cholera: A new homeland in Africa?' *American Journal of Tropical Medicine and Hygiene* 77: 705–13.
Gallo, W. (2008) *The Jolivert Safe Water for Families Project's Response to the Gonaives Floods*, Jolivert Safe Water for Families, Melbourne, FL.
Gupta, S.K. and Quick, R.E. (2006) 'Inadequate drinking water quality from tanker trucks following a tsunami disaster, Aceh, Indonesia, June 2005', *Disaster Prevention and Management* 15: 213–15.
Gupta, S.K., Suantio, A., Gray, A., Widyastuti, E., Jain, N., Rolos, R., Hoekstra, R.M. and Quick, R.E. (2007) 'Factors associated with *E. coli* contamination of household drinking water among tsunami and earthquake survivors, Indonesia', *American Journal of Tropical Medicine and Hygiene* 76: 1158–62.
Handzel, T. and Bamrah, S. (2006) *Trip Report: Evaluation of Pilot Intervention to Improve Household Drinking Water, Dong Thap Province, Vietnam*, Centers for Disease Control and Prevention, Altanta, GA.
Hoque, B.A. and Khanam, S. (Undated) *Efficiency and Effectiveness of Point-of Use Technologies in Emergency Drinking Water: An Evaluation of PUR and Aquatab in Rural Bangladesh*, Environment & Population Research Centre, Dhaka, Bangladesh.
IMC (2008) *The Gateway Initiative: Sensitizing Children to Promote Healthy Behaviors and Families*, International Medical Corps, Santa Monica, CA.
Johnston, R. (2008) *Preliminary Data: Response to Cyclone Sidr*, UNICEF, Dhaka, Bangladesh.
Lantagne, D. (2006) *Potters for Peace: Filter Production Facility Best Practices*, Potters for Peace, Managua, Nicaragua.
Lantagne, D. (2008) 'Sodium hypochlorite dosage for household and emergency water treatment', *Journal of the American Water Works Association* 100: 106–19.
Lantagne, D. (2009) *WASH Evidence Base/Knowledge Base and Data Collection Methodologies (EB/DCM) Workshop Rapporteur Report*, 26–29 January 2009. Geneva, Global WASH Cluster.
Mong, Y., Kaiser, R., Ibrahim, D., Rasoatiana, Razafimbololona, L. and Quick, R.E. (2001) 'Impact of the safe water system on water quality in cyclone-affected communities in Madagascar', *American Journal of Public Health* 91: 1577–79.
Noji, E.K. (ed.) (1997) *Public Health Consequences of Disasters*, Oxford University Press, New York.
Palmer, J. (2005) *Community Acceptability of Household Ceramic Water Filters Distributed during Oxfam's Response to the Tsunami in Sri Lanka*, London School of Hygiene and Tropical Medicine, London.
Ram, P.K., Blanton, E., Klinghoffer, D., Platek, M., Piper, J., Straif-Bourgeois, S., Bonner, M.R. and Mintz, E.D. (2007) 'Household water disinfection in hurricane-affected communities of Louisiana: Implications for disaster

preparedness for the general public', *American Journal of Public Health* 97 Suppl 1: S130–35.

Reller, M.E., Mong, Y.J., Hoekstra, R.M. and Quick, R.E. (2001) 'Cholera prevention with traditional and novel water treatment methods: An outbreak investigation in Fort-Dauphin, Madagascar', *American Journal of Public Health* 91: 1608–10.

Ritter, M. (2007) *Determinants of Adoption of Household Water Treatment in Haiti Jolivert Safe Water for Families (JSWF) Program*, Emory University, Atlanta, GA.

Roberts, L., Chartier, Y., Chartier, O., Malenga, G., Toole, M. and Rodka, H. (2001) 'Keeping clean water clean in a Malawi refugee camp: A randomized intervention trial', *Bulletin of the World Health Organization* 79: 280–87.

Schmidt, W.P. and Cairncross, S. (2009) 'Household water treatment in poor populations: Is there enough evidence for scaling up now?' *Environmental Science & Technology* 43: 986–92.

Scott, B., Curtis, V., Rabie, T. and Garbrah-Aidoo, N. (2007) 'Health in our hands, but not in our heads: Understanding hygiene motivation in Ghana', *Health Policy Plan* 22: 225–33.

Sobsey, M., Stauber, C.E., Casanova, L.M., Brown, J. and Elliott, M.A. (2008) 'Point of use household drinking water filtration: A practical, effective solution for providing sustained access to safe drinking water in the developing world', *Environmental Science & Technology* 42: 4261–67.

SP (2006) *PUR-Purifier of Water IDP Camp Distribution Program, Lira District, Northern Uganda, Project End Report*, Samaritan's Purse, Boone, NC.

Sphere (2004) *Humanitarian Charter and Minimum Standards in Disaster Response*, The Sphere Project, Geneva.

Toole, M. and Waldman, R.J. (1990) 'Prevention of excess mortality in refugee and displaced populations in developing countries', *JAMA* 263: 3296–302.

UNICEF (2007) *Demonstration Project: Investing in Safe Water for Children – PuR Pilot Application in Vietnam. Final Report to the United States Fund for UNICEF/ Procter & Gamble*, UNICEF Viet Nam Water, Environment & Sanitation (WES) Programme, Vietnam.

UNICEF/WHO (2008) *Progress on Drinking Water and Sanitation: Special Focus on Sanitation*, UNICEF/WHO, Geneva.

Walden, V.M., Lamond, E.A. and Field, S.A. (2005) 'Container contamination as a possible source of a diarrhoea outbreak in Abou Shouk camp, Darfur province, Sudan', *Disasters* 29: 213–21.

Watson, J., Gayer, M. and M, C. (2007) 'Epidemics after natural disasters', *Emerging Infectious Diseases* 13: 1–5.

WHO (2004) *Guidelines for Drinking-water Quality, 3rd Edition; Volume 1: Recommendations*, WHO, Geneva.

WHO (2005) *Household Water Treatment and Safe Storage Following Emergencies and Disasters*, World Health Organization, Geneva.

WHO (2008) *Guidelines for Drinking-water Quality: Second Addendum to Third Edition*, World Health Organization, Geneva.

Zehri, M. and Ensink, J.H. (2008) *Assessment of NeroxTM Water Treatment Device in Emergency Settings in Pakistan*, Oxfam and LSHTM, London.

CHAPTER 3

Water, sanitation, and hygiene in emergencies: summary review and recommendations for further research

Joe Brown, Sue Cavill, Oliver Cumming and Aurelie Jeandron

Abstract

Water, sanitation, and hygiene interventions can interrupt diarrhoeal disease transmission and reduce the burden of morbidity and mortality associated with faecal-oral infections. We know that rapid response of effective WASH infrastructure and services can prevent or lessen the impact of diarrhoeal outbreaks that can exacerbate the human suffering accompanying humanitarian crises. In this review summary, we present an overview of current knowledge about what works to prevent disease in emergency WASH response. We know that providing safe water, safe excreta disposal, and basic hygiene measures such as hand washing with soap are effective interventions both within emergency settings as well as in longer-term development, but innovation and further research are needed to make WASH response more effective. We propose key areas for critical research to support the evidence base for WASH interventions in emergencies and promote innovation.

Keywords: emergencies, humanitarian, water, sanitation, hygiene

Water, sanitation, and hygiene (WASH) measures are intended to protect health by reducing exposure to pathogens. Their implementation in non-emergency settings is supported by a wealth of evidence suggesting significant health gains as well as other benefits (Bartram and Cairncross, 2010). In emergency settings, rapid WASH provision can prevent outbreaks and an escalation of the total burden of disease and death associated with natural or man-made disasters. Outbreaks of diarrhoeal diseases, including dysentery and cholera, are common in emergencies. Faecal-oral diseases may account for more than 40 per cent of deaths in the acute phase of an emergency, with greater than 80 per cent of deaths in children under 2 years of age (Connolly et al., 2004). In some emergencies and post-emergency situations, diarrhoea can be responsible for the majority of deaths. During the Kurdish refugee crisis of 1991, for example, one estimate was that 70 per cent of total deaths were attributable to diarrhoea (including cholera) (Toole and Waldman, 1997). Post-response case studies and outbreak investigations have identified unsafe water (at source and point of use), lack of water (quantity), poor sanitation access or use, scarcity of soap and hand washing, and contaminated foods as risk factors for transmission. Kouadio et al. (2009) summarize infectious disease outbreaks following natural disasters and conflicts, many of which are directly related to WASH.

Emergency situations are challenging environments for WASH implementation, and recent experience from Haiti and elsewhere has highlighted the limitations of current emergency sanitation options (and to a lesser extent safe water supply and hygiene promotion) within humanitarian response (Shultz et al., 2009; Patel et al., 2011). The need for more suitable approaches and technologies for rapid deployment to emergencies has been widely acknowledged in the humanitarian sector and discussed at the recent Stoutenburg workshops (Johannessen, 2011).

The need for improved WASH strategies for emergencies has generated a number of new approaches that have been explored by relief organizations, leading to rapid innovation. However, there remains insufficient confidence and evidence of what works, what doesn't, and why in emerging processes, technologies, and approaches for humanitarian WASH services. Unknowns persist about which strategies are suitable for the immediate emergency phase and which technologies, practices, and approaches may permit a transition towards more sustainable solutions and future resilience.

We reviewed the existing guidance on best practice for WASH delivery in emergencies and published evidence on what works to control disease transmission. Based on our summary, we propose a number of areas for critical research to improve WASH response in humanitarian relief. This paper is an overview of this review.

Existing guidance: Best practice for wash interventions

There is an extensive grey literature outlining 'what works' and best practice in the delivery of WASH interventions in emergency settings, spanning intra-agency briefing notes, project reports, training packs, and lessons learnt or case study papers. Table 3.1 summarizes recommendations for best practice in the WASH response according to the widely cited Sphere Project (Sphere, 2011), and Table 3.2 illustrates the diversity of documents providing guidance for good practice in emergency response. Much of the knowledge about 'what works' is the mostly tacit knowledge held by the humanitarian workers who are mobilized in response and who learn on the job or by trial and error. Institutional memory is therefore diffuse and grows organically with additional experience from each crisis.

One of the challenges for practitioners seeking guidance has been the often diverse, and sometimes disparate, sources of information emerging from practitioners when this accumulated experience is communicated. Knowledge sharing has occurred not just through published papers but also through various sector forums – both online and traditional – as well as training and capacity-building activities held within and between operational agencies.

Table 3.1 Selected water, sanitation, and hygiene recommendations for emergency response

	Water		Sanitation		Hygiene
Standard	Indicators	Standard	Indicators	Standard	Indicators
Water quantity	Total basic water needs: 7.5–15 litres per day	**Environment free from human faeces**	All sanitation situated >30 m from any ground-water source	**Hygiene promotion implementation**	All facilities are appropriately used and maintained
	Max. distance to nearest water point <500 m; queuing time <30 min		Toilets are used (and children's faeces disposed of) hygienically		All wash hands after defecation/cleaning children, before eating/preparing food
Water quality	No faecal coliforms per 100 ml at point of delivery and use	**Appropriate and adequate toilet facilities**	Max. of 20 people use each toilet	**Identification and use of hygiene items**	All have access to hygiene items and these are used effectively
	No outbreak of water-borne or water-related diseases		Security threats are minimized, especially to women and girls		All women and girls of menstruating age are provided with appropriate menstrual hygiene materials
Water facilities	Household has min. 2 clean water collecting containers				
	At least 1 washing basin per 100 people				

Source: Sphere, 2011

Table 3.2 Selection of grey literature on WASH interventions in emergencies [all websites accessed 30 January 2012]

Type of document	Selected references	Link
Books and manuals	John Hopkins and IFRC (2008) *Public Health Guide for Emergencies,* 2nd edn	http://www.jhsph.edu/
	Davies, Jan and Robert Lambert (2002) *Engineering in Emergencies: A Practical Guide for Relief Workers,* Practical Action Publishing, Rugby	http://developmentbookshop.com
	MSF (1994) *Public Health Engineering in Emergency Situations*	
	ODI and A. Chalinder (1994) *Good Practice Reviews: Water and Sanitation in Emergencies*	http://www.odihpn.org/
	ACF International network (2005) *Water, Sanitation and Hygiene for Populations at Risk*	
Technical guidelines	Oxfam (2006) *Water Treatment Guidelines for Use in Emergencies*	http://www.oxfam.org.uk/
	House, S.J. and R.A. Reed (1997) *Emergency Water Sources: Guidelines for Selection and Treatment,* WEDC, Loughborough	
	ADPC (2000) *Tools and Resources for Post-disaster Relief*	
	IFRC (2008) *Household Water Treatment and Safe Storage in Emergencies*	http://www.ifrc.org/
Technical briefing notes	Oxfam (2010) *The Use of Poo Bags for Safe Excreta Disposal in Emergency Settings*	http://www.oxfam.org.uk/
	WHO and WEDC (2011) Technical notes for emergencies	http://wedc.lboro.ac.uk
	SuSanA (2009) *Sustainable Sanitation for Emergencies and Reconstruction Situations*	http://www.susana.org/
Conference proceedings	World Water Week (2009) *Abstracts volume, Workshop 5: Safe Water Service in Post-conflict and Post-disaster Context*	http://www.worldwaterweek.org/
	Oxfam working paper (1995) *Proceedings of an International Workshop: Sanitation in Emergency Situations*	http://www.oxfam.org.uk/
	P. Paul (2005) *31st WEDC International Conference, Proposals for a Rapidly Deployable Emergency Sanitation Treatment System*	http://www.wedc-knowledge.org
Lessons learned	ALNAP (2008) *Flood Disasters: Learning from Previous Relief and Recovery Operations*	http://www.alnap.org/resources/lessons.aspx
	Oxfam (2011) *Urban WASH Lessons Learned from Post-earthquake Response in Haiti*	http://www.oxfam.org.uk/

(continued)

Table 3.2 Selection of grey literature on WASH interventions in emergencies [all websites accessed 30 January 2012] (Continued)

Type of document	Selected references	Link
	UNICEF (2010) *Community Led Total Sanitation: Part of the Emergency Response in Flood-Affected Villages in Central Mozambique*	
Strategic documents	UNICEF (2010) *Core Commitments for Children in Humanitarian Action*	http://www.unicef.org
	Global WASH Cluster, Strategic Plan 2011–2015	
	WELL (2006) *A Strategic Approach to Water and Sanitation in Disasters*	http://www.wedc-knowledge.org
Websites	WEDC publications	http://wedc.lboro.ac.uk
	WASH cluster website	http://washcluster.net
	Tearfund International Learning Zone	http://tilz.tearfund.org

Note: Acronyms: IFRC, International Federation of the Red Cross and Red Crescent Societies; MSF, Médecins Sans Frontières; ODI, Overseas Development Institute; ACF, Action Contre la Faim; ADPC, Asian Disasters Preparedness Centre; ALNAP, Active Learning Network for Accountability and Performance in Humanitarian Action; WHO, World Health Organization; WEDC, Water, Engineering and Development Centre; SuSanA, Sustainable Sanitation Alliance; UNICEF, United Nations Children's Fund.

Technical enquiry services, for example those offered by RedR, Practical Action, DEW Point, and KnowledgePoint, have played an important role in responding to ad hoc requests for guidance.

Some agencies, particularly international NGOs and UN agencies, have published conference proceedings, technical guidance manuals, and other documents in order to share knowledge. Much of the best practice literature has historically reflected in-agency policy rather than broader sector-level consensus but has laid important foundations for inter-agency dialogue.

There have been various communities of practice and inter-agency meetings convened over the last 20 years to share learning and ideas. Perhaps the most significant recent initiative was the establishment of the WASH Cluster. The 'cluster approach' was one pillar of the reforms agreed in 2006 by UN agencies and other organizations active in the field of humanitarian response. The WASH Cluster has three key responsibilities: 1) setting standard and policy; 2) building response capacity; and 3) providing operational support. Under the first objective of standard setting, the WASH Cluster seeks to both consolidate and disseminate standards and to identify best practice. The cluster has played an important role in both providing a platform for the sharing of learning, and providing a source of information for those seeking guidance through its website.

Another more formalized attempt to improve guidance within the sector is the Sphere project and its *Sphere Handbook*, now in its third edition

(Sphere, 2011). Rooted in a rights-based and people-centred approach, the *Sphere Handbook* provides minimum standards for humanitarian responses across six sectors, including WASH. The guidelines are the result of 'sector-wide consultations ... involving a wide range of agencies, organizations and individuals, including governments and United Nations' and are generally accepted by the humanitarian sector as representing 'best practice'. Table 3.1 summarizes the key standards and examples of the recommended indicators from the Sphere Project.

Inclusion

Whilst there are examples of good practice, it should be noted that there is no systematic approach or guidelines to issues of inclusiveness in the emergency context. The WASH response should be inclusive with respect to:

Women and girls. Safety concerns of women and girls have been documented challenges to implementing sanitation in a humanitarian context (Atuyambe et al., 2011), and females are also usually responsible for managing water, protecting water quality, and maintaining domestic hygiene. Water provision, water quality interventions, and hygiene promotion in an emergency setting must focus on women and girls, include their active participation and empowerment, and account for their needs and preferences in response strategies (Nawaz et al., 2010). Although guidelines for meeting menstrual hygiene needs exist (e.g. Sphere standards), more work is needed to characterize appropriate strategies to meet needs (Sommer, Chapter 5).

People with disabilities. The World Bank estimates that 20 per cent of the world's poorest people are disabled, yet little attention has been paid to the needs for unrestricted access to WASH. This is especially true in the humanitarian context. Innovation for sanitation access must include careful consideration of meeting the needs of people with disabilities. Some refugee and displaced persons populations may have a high percentage of people with disabilities, and this may be especially true after natural disasters that have resulted in bodily harm (Wolbring, 2011).

Children. Children need different excreta disposal facilities depending on age. If nappies are distributed, waste management is an issue; however with non-disposable nappies there is the problem of washing. Providing potties for children is an option where children are afraid of falling into a pit latrine or might not want to use a toilet for other reasons such as darkness, snakes and other animals, the smell, and dirtiness. Few sanitation options have been documented specifically for use by children, although they are among the most susceptible group to faecal-oral disease.

People living with HIV/AIDS. Populations affected by HIV/AIDS are especially susceptible to WASH-related illnesses and appropriate WASH responses may need to consider this and other vulnerable populations in response; high levels of HIV itself can lead to interruption in WASH services and increased vulnerability to disease (Moss, 2004).

Review of published evidence: water supply and quality

There is strong evidence that both sufficient water (quantity) and safety (quality) are critical to interrupting disease transmission in humanitarian settings. Better models are needed for rapid delivery of water to dispersed populations and more research is needed to support adherence to water quality interventions.

There are established and accepted methods for water provision in emergencies (e.g. Sherlock, 1988) although context-specific factors such as political, economic, social, and environmental constraints may impact how these are put into place (Shelley, 1994), how effective they are, and whether they may result in increased risk of vector-borne diseases such as malaria or dengue (Bayoh et al., 2011). Installation may be complex, requiring special expertise, and time-consuming, slowing response time and the delivery of safe drinking water in the critical early stages of response. The pursuit of more sustainable water supplies in the first instance may delay response time but may have longer-term advantages (Randall et al., 2008). The process of selecting from available technologies itself may not be straightforward in rapid response, where there is a need for immediate access to potable drinking water but acknowledgement that the supply needs to be sustainable. The need for immediate water provision often takes precedence, justifiably. The delayed water supply response following the 1999 earthquake in Turkey, for example, was linked to higher faecal-oral disease seroconversion in children (Sencan et al., 2004).

There is evidence that sufficient water (quantity) for health and well-being, including hygiene needs, is protective against disease in emergency settings, and international standards exist for water provision in emergencies (Table 3.1). Cronin et al. (2008) observed that households reporting diarrhoea within the previous 24 hours had a mean 26 per cent less water available. In a seven-country review of 51 camps from 1998 to 2000, Spiegel et al. (2002) concluded that camps with lower than the recommended 15 litres of water per person per day had significantly higher under-five mortality in a systematic risk factor analysis. Following the arrival of 800,000 Rwandan refugees into the Democratic Republic of the Congo in 1994, 85 per cent of the first month's 50,000 deaths were due to diarrhoeal diseases (cholera and shigellosis). The primary risk factor was lack of access to water: the per capita water allowance was 0.2 L per day in the first week of the crisis (Connolly et al., 2004). Further, water that is supplied must be accessible and acceptable to users. Atuyambe et al. (2011) found that the inconsistent nature of tanked water provision as well as taste acceptability issues resulted in camp residents using untreated surface water. This also underscores the importance of prior knowledge about water safety among the population being served. Water supplies must be both safe and acceptable to users, although quantity may take precedence over quality (Luff, 2004) in terms of delivering a wide range of health benefits, including those that are primarily linked to hygiene.

There is some evidence that community ownership of water supplies and demand-driven approaches may increase the sustainability of water supplies

(Boydell, 1999), but how anything but a top-down, supply-side solution for water provision can be effected in an emergency situation is unclear. In many cases, there would be ethical obstacles to requiring community investment in these types of situation. Transition to a longer-term, sustainable approach to water supply following an emergency often requires a change of approach. Solutions that are both rapidly deployable and come with a plan for the transition to long-term sustainability are needed, especially if new systems and services make communities more resilient against future emergencies. The management of water supplies in post-emergency transition has received some attention (e.g. Pinera and Reed, 2009), but the well-known institutional, financial, environmental, and social constraints that limit water infrastructure services in low-income settings threaten access to safe water once any special attention (funding, human resources) that may have been the result of an emergency has been redirected.

Water quality interventions (point-of-use treatment and safe storage)

There is evidence that drinking water quality at the point of consumption is an important determinant of risk of disease, so a number of studies have focused on point-of-use (POU) water quality in humanitarian response (Clasen and Boisson, 2006; Gupta et al., 2007; Steele et al., 2008). Water quality interventions such as POU water treatment and safe storage have been studied for their effectiveness in reducing risk of diarrhoeal diseases (including cholera) in emergency response and refugee camp situations. Current evidence is suggestive of protective effects of both active treatment and safe water storage (such as narrow-mouth containers or containers with controlled access) with documented effects against cholera (Hatch et al., 1994; Reller et al., 2001; Hashizume et al., 2008; Shultz et al., 2009) and all diarrhoeal diseases (Roberts, 2001; Kunii et al., 2002; Mourad, 2004; Walden et al., 2005; Doocy and Burnham, 2006; Hashizume et al., 2008). Chlorination, chlorination preceded by flocculation, boiling, and ceramic filters have been studied. Work by Lantagne (2011) has shown that the use of POU water quality interventions in emergencies has the greatest likelihood of success when effective technologies are distributed to households with contaminated water who are familiar and comfortable with the option before the emergency, and have the training and support necessary to use the option after the emergency.

Critically, consistency of use or adherence may limit the impact of POU water treatment, and some evidence for low adherence exists from studies conducted in humanitarian response. Mong et al. (2001) reported 50 per cent adherence to POU chlorination and Clasen and Boisson reported approximately the same level of adherence to POU ceramic candle filtration at 16 weeks post-implementation. Colindres et al. (2007) reported 45 per cent adherence to a POU combined flocculent-disinfectant at 3 weeks after distribution. Atuyambe et al. (2011) reported 'unsuccessful' uptake of boiling in Uganda due to taste acceptability issues in the target population. Water quality interventions can only protect public health if they are used correctly and consistently, and adherence is especially important when the risk of disease associated with untreated water is high.

Research needs: Water supply and water quality

Research is needed to modify or develop technologies for rapid distribution in emergencies so that beneficiaries in dispersed emergency situations have faster, more predictable, and longer-lasting access to safer drinking water. This includes both rapid deployment of drinking water treatment and distribution methods for safeguarding water to the POU. Because safe water may be distributed and subject to recontamination, appropriate distribution methods to the POU with a focus on protecting water quality are needed. Dedicated safe storage containers or packaged water distribution may be needed to safeguard quality. The challenge of rapidly providing 15+ litres per person per day of safe water (and the means to protect it from recontamination) is formidable.

Also, more research is needed on appropriate means of creating high adherence to POU water treatment and safe storage through effective technology design and behaviour change. The available evidence from POU interventions in the humanitarian context suggests that water quality interventions may be protective against disease but high adherence is probably required to maintain health impact. A number of studies of POU water treatment from non-emergency settings have shown reduced use of interventions over time, raising questions about the potential for sustained use (Luby et al., 2001; Brown et al., 2007; Mausezahl et al., 2009) and therefore health impact when untreated water is unsafe.

Review of published evidence: Sanitation

Effective sanitation can prevent disease and rapid response is important. Whilst basic options exist, innovation is needed to meet known challenges.

Safe excreta disposal is the first line of defence against faecal-oral pathogen transmission. Sanitation options for the humanitarian context have been widely studied and it is widely recognized that no one solution is appropriate for all cases (Howard, 1996; Wisner and Adams, 2002; Harvey and Reed, 2005). Excreta need to be contained in the quickest time possible to prevent the spread of infection (Sencan et al., 2004), but currently available options may not be adequate to meet the challenge of rapid response. Some emerging sanitation solutions are not developed or refined enough to be available for immediate dispatch in the first phase of an emergency.

Sanitation is often a defecation field, trench latrine, or communal latrine solution until the immediate emergency phase is over, during which capacity is quickly overwhelmed by the numbers of users, pits fill up and become a hazard, and maintaining hygienic conditions becomes a challenge. Open defecation, and the use of plastic bags (flying latrines) are commonly practised alternatives (Patel et al., 2011). Lora-Suarez et al. (2002) noted a significant increase in giardiasis among children associated with shared sanitation (compared with individual household sanitation) following an earthquake in Colombia. Standards recommend no more than 20 people per latrine (Table 3.1), but for maintaining hygienic conditions one household per latrine is ideal.

Problems with safe excreta disposal were particularly evident in Haiti (Johannessen, 2011; Bastable and Lamb, Chapter 7). The inability to dig pit latrines – due to a high water table, concrete sites, or lack of permission – slowed the aid effort considerably. Agencies took many days, if not weeks, to construct wooden raised latrines with small holding tanks. In 2009 similar problems were experienced in the floods in Greater Manila, the Philippines. The use of Portaloos as a temporary measure in these contexts proved inadequate owing to high cost and small storage capacity. Such examples illustrate that agencies may be poorly equipped to deal with the rapid provision of safe excreta disposal in urban emergency contexts.

Research needs: Sanitation

Wastewater and faecal sludge treatment and disposal. There is a clear need for innovation in managing wastewater and faecal sludges that are generated in the humanitarian context. Innovative, decentralized wastewater treatment options (membrane bioreactors, constructed wetlands, anaerobic filters) have been studied (e.g. Paul, 2005; Randall et al., 2008) but have not been widely adopted. Current solutions for sludges, such as desludging and sludge disposal and treatment kits, may be too costly and require skilled management, and may result in health risks where the sludge is finally dumped. There has been some innovation with desludging (Oxfam GB's work with diaphragm mud pumps, supernatant water pump), but more work remains to be done to drive down costs and expand the range of appropriate, practical options. Where and how waste is disposed of is critically important to containing faecal-oral disease (Howard, 1996).

Containment and chemical disinfection of waste and wastewater from cholera- and other infectious disease-impacted environments has been practised using chlorine, lime, and other means, although the effectiveness of these strategies *in situ* in reducing target microbial contaminants has not been formally assessed and deserves greater attention.

Sanitation under challenging conditions. Implementing effective excreta containment under challenging physical conditions such as unstable soils, high water tables, and in flood-prone areas remains a challenge in both the development and the post-emergency context (Djonoputro et al., 2010). Alternative systems may be required, including lining of pits to prevent pits from collapsing or building raised latrines (when digging down is not an option). There is potential to develop new technologies (such as septic tanks that can be rapidly constructed in areas with a high water table) as well as a need for more research on the effect of existing and emerging strategies for sanitation on available water sources.

Some settings may require unconventional approaches. Technical solutions need to be innovative and responsive to the specific physical, social, and cultural circumstances of the disaster-affected population. There has been some experience with people using a Peepoo bag (a double bag system containing powdered urea which prevents bad smells and speeds up the biodigestion process) or simple biodegradable bags (Patel et al., 2011), although more research is needed to characterize the role of Peepoo or conventional bags in meeting emergency sanitation needs and their implications for sludge treatment and disposal.

Design. Some sanitation options may benefit from design improvements for specific contexts. Plastic sheeting as a superstructure material, used in rapid response, often gets ripped, which has implications for dignity and security and often means the latrine isn't used (Johannessen, 2011). Oxfam has done some innovative work with prefabricated superstructure(s) that can be shipped or easily assembled with local materials and easily erected over latrines on site. Sanitation options that are user-friendly for women, men, children, and disabled persons exist, but innovation may increase available options' acceptability, effectiveness in excreta containment, safety, and maintenance over time. This is an area of rapid development by sectoral stakeholders, but focused research is needed to evaluate and implement emerging options.

Review of published evidence: Hygiene

The role of hand washing in preventing faecal-oral disease transmission is known, including in outbreaks. Promotion of hand washing with soap involves behaviour change, which can be slow. Are there rapid approaches that work? Is there a role for hardware?

Hygiene interventions can interrupt faecal-oral disease transmission and hand washing with soap in particular may be critical in outbreaks. Peterson et al. (1998) demonstrated that regular soap distribution (240 g bar soap per person per month) resulted in a 27 per cent reduction in diarrhoeal disease among households with consistent soap availability in a refugee camp in Malawi, and two studies have suggested a protective effect of hand washing with soap against cholera in outbreaks (Reller et al., 2001; Hutin et al., 2003). Soap availability and use behaviour is also critical, however, and user preferences and knowledge must be addressed, as suggested by data from a Ugandan emergency response in 2010 (Atuyambe et al., 2011) where hand washing was limited by soap type preferences and inconsistent availability. These factors suggest that hygiene promotion in emergencies is recommended and should accompany soap provision. There are examples of innovative hygiene promotion approaches such as Community Health Clubs that have been promoted in IDP camps in Uganda. No peer-reviewed studies exist on the associated hygiene 'hardware' such as hand washing stations or hygiene kits that may promote healthy hygiene behaviours in an emergency context. Rapidly deployable hardware that may aid in hygiene promotion is an area of potentially important innovation for WASH emergency response.

Research needs: Hygiene

Hygiene hardware innovation and research may facilitate more effective behaviour change. Hand washing stations or personal hygiene kits may increase uptake and consistency of hand washing. Their use in humanitarian response should be formally assessed.

Hygiene promotion software that rapidly increases hand washing and healthy hygiene behaviours should be the focus of innovation and evaluation. Soap distribution may need to be supplemented by specific supporting activities to be most effective. Given the critical role of hand hygiene in protecting health – especially during an outbreak – hand washing behaviours may merit further research to make the available interventions more effective.

The need for more research

Within the humanitarian emergency sector, the importance of the research and evidence base is well recognized. There is a culture that is supportive of research as well as key champions together with the motivation to undertake further research. NGOs and operational agencies (such as Oxfam, ACF, MSF, Tearfund, IRC, and IFRC) are proactively innovating in humanitarian response technologies and appropriate WASH product design, either individually or with inter-agency cooperation. They are working closely with product designers and suppliers to generate new technologies for rapid deployment in humanitarian settings. Experience has shown that the outputs of research – technologies, techniques, and processes – tend to be rapidly adopted.

There is a need to investigate innovative relief support services, tools, and technologies for water, sanitation, and hygiene (WASH) regionally and globally to meet the needs of disaster-affected communities in a modern context and deliver solutions at scale. The WASH response must be rapid to be effective: outbreaks happen quickly. Whilst there are kit-based and other rapidly deployable solutions (particularly for water), this is an area that deserves further research and innovation to improve response time post-emergency. Few WASH agencies currently stockpile standardized kits, even though kits are probably necessary to achieve rapid response.

Incorporating applied research into emergency response and publishing the results can help accelerate innovation. Most disaster response experience related to water, sanitation, and hygiene is not recorded in the peer-reviewed literature: communication of findings in the form of peer-reviewed research or case studies is understandably a second consideration after more immediate needs are met. Moreover, crisis situations themselves are often not suited to controlled research, and experimental methods may not be applied for ethical, logistical, financial, or human resource reasons. Therefore, few experimental studies of WASH interventions are conducted in humanitarian settings. Nevertheless, there is an urgent need to learn more about how to do research in this context, and the implications of different methods for the rigour of research in emergencies and thus the reliability of the evidence. Of the available observational and retrospective studies, case studies are most common and report context-specific data on acceptability, use, and impact of strategies employed. Whilst such studies are useful as 'snapshots' of the success of available practice, they may be more a commentary on the operational and programmatic responses to specific emergency situations themselves rather than controlled experiments of specific WASH interventions. Communication of findings is critical to collective learning about what works in WASH response.

Conclusion and recommendations

Evidence suggests that providing safe water, safe excreta disposal, and basic hygiene measures such as hand washing are effective interventions both within emergency settings and in longer-term development. Recent experience from humanitarian relief suggests progress has still to be made in meeting the basic WASH needs of people in crisis, however. We propose the following immediate priorities for research and innovation:

- *Innovative sanitation options for difficult settings.* To identify and/or develop new emergency kits that are appropriate to a number of difficult settings including: high water tables, urban settings, and unstable soil situations (Bastable and Lamb, Chapter 7). In addition improved promotional messaging is required for rapid take up of the facilities. Work in this area is expected to fill an important gap in understanding the solutions required in both *in situ* and displaced situations including in dense/urban and scattered contexts.
- *Technologies for water provision for dispersed communities.* Whilst there is an abundance of technologies available for bulk water treatment for rapid provision of clean water in emergencies, the picture is less clear when it comes to providing water for dispersed affected populations (Johannessen, 2011; Bastable and Lamb, Chapter 7; Luff and Dorea, Chapter 6). There is a need to modify or develop technologies for rapid distribution in dispersed emergency situations to ensure faster, more predictable, and longer-lasting access to safe drinking water.
- *Approaches to promote consistent, correct, and sustained use of water quality interventions.* Point-of-use (POU) water treatment and safe storage has been shown to be effective and suitable for rapid access to safe water in relief settings (Lantagne and Clasen, Chapter 2). Documented low adherence may, however, limit the protective effects of these interventions. More research is needed on whether new technologies, new approaches, or new behaviour change interventions – or more likely a combination of all three – may play a role in providing sustained access to safer water at the point of consumption.
- *Effective hygiene hardware and software.* Hand washing stations, safe water in sufficient quantity, and the availability of soap can contribute to more

effective hygiene. Rapidly deployable hand washing stations have not been systematically evaluated in a humanitarian setting. As for POU, further research is required to assess whether and how new technologies, new approaches, or new behaviour-change interventions may increase the uptake of hand washing as a sustained practice in the relief context.

Emergency response happens within the longer-term development process (Davis, 1988) and WASH strategies that promote or are consistent with sustainable development over time are needed. Institutional memory of organizations is an important factor in ensuring appropriate response in emergency settings, since programmatic lessons learned may help improve WASH response (Anema and Fesselet, 2003). Also, many refugee or displaced persons camps are in existence for long periods, up to many years (e.g. Sudan, Palestine: Mourad, 2004; Walden et al., 2005). Although this subject is too big to deal with adequately in this paper, it is one that requires further research.

About the authors

Joe Brown (joebrown@lshtm.ac.uk) was at the time of writing an environmental engineer and lecturer at the London School of Hygiene and Tropical Medicine. He is now Assistant Professor at the School of Civil and Environmental Engineering at Georgia Institute of Technology. **Sue Cavill** is the SHARE Research Manager based at WaterAid. At the time of writing, **Oliver Cumming** was the Policy Research Manager for the SHARE consortium based at LSHTM. He is now a Lecturer at LSHTM. **Aurelie Jeandron** is the SHARE Research Assistant based at LSHTM.

The authors – Sue Cavill in particular – would like to thank Andy Bastable (Oxfam) and David Woolnough, John Adlam and Brenda Coughlan (DFID) whose experience, inspiration, ideas, and collaboration led to the development of this paper.

References

Anema, A. and Fesselet, J.F. (2003) 'A volcanic issue: Lessons learned in Goma', *Waterlines* 21: 9–11.

Atuyambe, L.M., Ediau, M., Orach, C.G., Musenero, M. and Bazeyo, W. (2011) 'Land slide disaster in eastern Uganda: Rapid assessment of water, sanitation and hygiene situation in Bulucheke camp, Bududa district', *Environmental Health: A Global Access Science Source* 10: 38.

Bartram, J. and Cairncross, S. (2010) 'Hygiene, sanitation, and water: Forgotten foundations of health', *PLoS Medicine* 7: e1000367.

Bastable, A. and Lamb, J. (2015) 'Innovative designs and approaches in sanitation for challenging and complex humanitarian urban contexts', Water, Sanitation and Hygiene in Humanitarian Contexts, Practical Action Publishing, Rugby, UK. <http://dx.doi.org/10.3362/9781780448831.007>.

Bayoh, M.N., Akhwale, W., Ombok, M., Sang, D., Enoki, S.C., Koros, D., Walker, E.D., Williams, H.A., Burke, H., Armstrong, G.L., Cetron, M.S., Weinberg,

M., Breiman, R. & Hamel, M.J. (2011) 'Malaria in Kakuma refugee camp, Turkana, Kenya: Facilitation of *Anopheles arabiensis* vector populations by installed water distribution and catchment systems', *Malaria Journal* 10: 149.

Boydell, R.A. (1999) 'Making rural water supply and sanitation projects sustainable', *Waterlines* 18: 2–4.

Brown, J., Sobsey, M.D. and Proum, S. (2007) *Use of Ceramic Water Filters in Cambodia*, WSP-World Bank Field Note, Washington, DC.

Clasen, T. and Boisson, S. (2006) 'Household-based ceramic water filters for the treatment of drinking water in disaster response: An assessment of a pilot programme in the Dominican Republic', *Water Practice & Technology* <http://www.iwaponline.com/wpt/001/wpt0010031.htm>

Colindres, R.E., Jain, S., Bowen, A., Mintz, E. & Domond, P. (2007) 'After the flood: An evaluation of in-home drinking water treatment with combined flocculent-disinfectant following Tropical Storm Jeanne: Gonaives, Haiti, 2004', *Journal of Water & Health* 5: 367–74.

Connolly, M.A., Gayer, M., Ryan, M.J., Salama, P., Spiegel, P. and Heymann, D.L. (2004) 'Communicable diseases in complex emergencies: Impact and challenges', *Lancet* 364: 1974–83.

Cronin, A.A., Shrestha, D., Cornier, N., Abdulla, F., Ezard, N. and Aramburu, C. (2008) 'A review of water and sanitation provision in refugee camps in association with selected health and nutrition indicators: The need for integrated service provision', *Journal of Water and Health* 6: 1–13.

Davis, J. (1988) 'From emergency relief to long-term water development', *Waterlines* 6: 29–31.

Djonoputro, E.R., Blackett, I., Rosenboom, J.W. and Weitz, A. (2010) 'Understanding sanitation options in challenging environments', *Waterlines* 29: 186–203.

Doocy, S. & Burnham, G. (2006) 'Point-of-use water treatment and diarrhoea reduction in the emergency context: An effectiveness trial in Liberia', *Tropical Medicine and International Health* 11: 1542–52.

Gupta, S.K., Suantio, A., Gray, A., Widyastuti, E., Jain, N., Rolos, R., Hoekstra, R.M. & Quick, R. (2007) 'Factors associated with *E. coli* contamination of household drinking water among tsunami and earthquake survivors, Indonesia', *American Journal of Tropical Medicine & Hygiene* 76: 1158–62.

Harvey, P.A. & Reed, R.A. (2005) 'Planning environmental sanitation programmes in emergencies', *Disasters* 29: 129–51.

Hashizume, M., Wagatsuma, Y., Faruque, A.S., Hayashil, T., Hunter, P.R., Armstrong, B. and Sack, D.A. (2008) 'Factors determining vulnerability to diarrhoea during and after severe floods in Bangladesh', *Journal of Water & Health* 6: 323–32.

Hatch, D.L., Waldman, R.J., Lungu, G.W. and Piri, C. (1994) 'Epidemic cholera during refugee resettlement in Malawi', *International Journal of Epidemiology* 23: 1292–9.

Howard, J. (1996) 'Rethinking the unthinkable effective excreta disposal in emergency situations', *Waterlines* 15: 5–6.

Hutin, Y., Luby, S. and Paquet, C. (2003) 'A large cholera outbreak in Kano City, Nigeria: The importance of hand washing with soap and the danger of street-vended water', *Journal of Water & Health* 1: 45–52.

Johannessen, A. (2011) 'Identifying gaps in emergency sanitation: Design of new kits to increase effectiveness in emergencies', 2 day workshop, 22–23 February 2011, Stoutenburg, Netherlands.

Kouadio, K.I., Kamigaki, T. & Oshitani, H. (2009) 'Strategies for communicable diseases response after disasters in developing countries' (Special Issue: Our social activities are always related to outbreaks of infectious diseases), *Journal of Disaster Research* 4: 298–308.

Kunii, O., Nakamura, S., Abdur, R. & Wakai, S. (2002) 'The impact on health and risk factors of the diarrhoea epidemics in the 1998 Bangladesh floods', *Public Health* 116: 68–74.

Lantagne, D. (2011) *Household Water Treatment and Safe Storage in Emergencies*, PhD thesis, London School of Hygiene and Tropical Medicine.

Lantagne, D. and Clasen, T. (2012) 'Point-of-use water treatment in emergency response', *Waterlines* 31.

Lora-Suarez, F., Marin-Vazquez, C., Loango, N., Gallego, M., Torres, E., Gonzales, M.M., Castano-Osorio, J.C. and Gome-Marin, J.E. (2002) 'Giardiasis in children living in post-earthquake camps from Armenia (Colombia)', *BMC Public Health* 2: 5.

Luby, S., Agboatwalla, M., Raza, A., Sobel, J., Mintz, E., Baier, K., Rahbar, M., Qureshi, S., Hassan, R., Ghouri, F., Hoekstra, R.M. and Gangarosa, E. (2001) 'A low-cost intervention for cleaner drinking water in Karachi, Pakistan', *International Journal of Infectious Diseases* 5: 144–50.

Luff, R. (2004) 'Paying too much for purity? Development of more appropriate emergency water treatment methods', in *People-centered Approaches to Water and Environmental Sanitation, WEDC International Conference*, 2004 Vientiane, Lao PDR.

Mausezahl, D., Christen, A., Pacheco, G.D., Alvarez Tellez, F., Iriarte, M., Zapata, M.E., Cevallos, M., Hattendorf, J., Cattaneo, M.D., Arnold, B., Smith, T.A. and Colford, J.M. Jr (2009) 'Solar drinking water disinfection (SODIS) to reduce childhood diarrhoea in rural Bolivia: A cluster-randomized, controlled trial', *PLoS Medicine* 6: e1000125.

Mong, Y., Kaiser, R., Ibrahim, D., Rasoatiana, Razafimbololona, L. & Quick, R.E. (2001) 'Impact of the safe water system on water quality in cyclone-affected communities in Madagascar', *American Journal of Public Health* 91: 1577–9.

Moss, S. (2004) '"Complex drought' in southern Africa: A water and sanitation perspective', *Waterlines* 22: 19–21.

Mourad, T.A.A. (2004) 'Palestinian refugee conditions associated with intestinal parasites and diarrhoea: Nuseirat refugee camp as a case study', *Public Health* 118: 131–42.

Nawaz, J., Lal, S., Raza, S. and House, S. (2010) 'Oxfam experience of providing screened toilet, bathing and menstruation units in its earthquake response in Pakistan', *Gender & Development* 18: 81–86.

Patel, D., Brooks, N. & Bastable, A. (2011) 'Excreta disposal in emergencies: Bag and Peepoo trials with internally displaced people in Port-au-Prince', *Waterlines* 30: 61–77.

Paul, P. (2005) 'Proposals for a rapidly deployable emergency sanitation treatment system', in Kayaga, S. (ed.), *Maximizing the Benefits from Water and Environmental Sanitation: 31st WEDC Conference, Kampala, Uganda*. Water, Engineering and Development Centre (WEDC), Loughborough University of Technology, Loughborough.

Peterson, E.A., Roberts, L., Toole, M.J. and Peterson, D.E. (1998) 'The effect of soap distribution on diarrhoea: Nyamithuthu Refugee Camp', *International Journal of Epidemiology* 27: 520–4.

Pinera, J.F. and Reed, R.A. (2009) 'A tale of two cities: Restoring water services in Kabul and Monrovia', *Disasters* 33: 574–90.

Randall, J.J., Navaratne, A., Rand, E.C. and Hagos, Y. (2008) 'Integrating environmental sustainability into the water and sanitation sector: Lessons from tsunami disaster response', in *Proceedings of the 33rd WEDC International Conference Access to Sanitation and Safe Water: Global Partnerships and Local Actions, Accra, Ghana*.

Reller, M.E., Mong, Y.J., Hoekstra, R.M. and Quick, R.E. (2001) 'Cholera prevention with traditional and novel water treatment methods: An outbreak investigation in Fort-Dauphin, Madagascar', *American Journal of Public Health* 91: 1608–10.

Roberts, L., Chartier, Y., Chartier, O., Malenga, G., Toole, M. & Rodka, H. (2001) 'Keeping clean water clean in a Malawi refugee camp: A randomized intervention trial', *Bulletin of the World Health Organization* 79: 280–87.

Sencan, I., Sahin, I., Kaya, D., Oksuz, S. & Yildirim, M. (2004) 'Assessment of HAV and HEV seroprevalence in children living in post-earthquake camps from Duzce, Turkey', *European Journal of Epidemiology* 19: 461–5.

Shelley, C. (1994) 'Refugee water supplies: Some political considerations', *Waterlines* 13: 4–6.

Sherlock, P. (1988) 'Coping with equipment in emergencies', *Waterlines* 6: 26–28.

Shultz, A., Omollo, J.O., Burke, H., Qassim, M., Ochieng, J.B., Weinberg, M., Feikin, D.R. and Breiman, R.F. (2009) 'Cholera outbreak in Kenyan refugee camp: Risk factors for illness and importance of sanitation', *American Journal of Tropical Medicine & Hygiene* 80: 640–5.

Sphere Project (2011) *The Sphere Handbook: Humanitarian Charter and Minimum Standards in Humanitarian Response*, Sphere, Practical Action Publishing, Rugby, UK. http://www.developmentbookshelf.com/doi/book/10.3362/9781908176202 [accessed 22nd May 2015 http://www.developmentbookshelf.com/doi/book/10.3362/9781908176202 [Accessed 22nd May 2015 <http:/dx.doi.org/10.3362/9781908176202>.

Sommer, M. (2012) 'Menstrual hygiene management in humanitarian emergencies: Gaps and Recommendations', in *Water, Sanitation and Hygiene in Humanitarian Contexts*, Practical Action Publishing, Rugby, UK. <http://dx.doi.org/10.3362/9781780448831.005>

Spiegel, P., Sheik, M., Gotway-Crawford, C. and Salama, P. (2002) 'Health programmes and policies associated with decreased mortality in displaced people in postemergency phase camps: A retrospective study', *Lancet* 360: 1927–34.

Steele, A., Clarke, B. and Watkins, O. (2008) 'Impact of jerry can disinfection in a camp environment: Experiences in an IDP camp in Northern Uganda', *Journal of Water and Health* 6: 559–64.

Toole, M.J. and Waldman, R.J. (1997) 'The public health aspects of complex emergencies and refugee situations', *Annual Review of Public Health* 18: 283–312.

Walden, V.M., Lamond, E.A. and Field, S.A. (2005) 'Container contamination as a possible source of a diarrhoea outbreak in Abou Shouk camp, Darfur province, Sudan' (Special Issue: Food security in complex emergencies), *Disasters* 29: 213–21.

Wisner, B. and Adams, J. (2002) *Environmental Health in Emergencies and Disasters: A Practical Guide*, World Health Organization, Geneva.

Wolbring, G. (2011) 'Disability, displacement and public health: A vision for Haiti', *Canadian Journal of Public Health* 102: 157–59.

CHAPTER 4
Water and wastes in the context of the West African Ebola outbreak: turning uncertain science into pragmatic guidance in Sierra Leone

Richard C. Carter, J. Peter Dumble, St John Day, and Michael Cowing

Abstract

In 2014–15 the three West African countries of Guinea, Sierra Leone and Liberia experienced the largest Ebola outbreak then on record. As Ebola care facilities were established throughout Sierra Leone, guidance was required regarding the management of liquid and solid wastes (including clinical wastes), and regarding the protection of water resources around the care facilities. In drafting the guidance, the authors of this paper had to take into account a number of key scientific, institutional capacity and public perception issues. As a consequence of its geology, climate and poor sanitation Sierra Leone may be especially vulnerable to groundwater pollution via rapid flow paths from the surface to shallow water tables. The guidance documents (Ministry of Health and Sanitation (2015) Waste management at Ebola care facilities*; Ministry of Water Resources (2015)* Protection of water resources from wastes at and around Ebola care facilities*) had to simplify and communicate a body of uncertain science; and they had to recognize the limited resources and capacities nationally for managing wastes and protecting water resources. The authors nevertheless attempted to provide pragmatic and useable approaches.*

Keywords: Ebola; waste water treatment; solid waste disposal; sanitation

Introduction

The first case of Ebola virus disease (for brevity referred to in this paper simply as Ebola) in West Africa was reported in Guinea in March 2014. The infection quickly spread to large numbers of victims in Guinea, Sierra Leone and Liberia, with much smaller numbers in Nigeria, Mali and Senegal. By the end of March 2015 the cumulative case count in the three worst-affected countries had exceeded 25,000, with more than 10,000 deaths (WHO, 2015).

Prior to 2014, no outbreak of Ebola had come close to the scale of the crisis in West Africa. The largest previous outbreak involved 425 cases in Uganda in the year 2000. Out of 24 documented outbreaks between 1976 and 2012, the average number of cases per outbreak was just under 100. The average fatality rate was 67 per cent (all data from WHO, 2014a).

On the basis of reported cases and deaths in the 2014–15 West African outbreak, Sierra Leone was the worst affected of the three intense-transmission countries, experiencing nearly half the reported cases and about 35 per cent of the documented deaths (WHO, 2015). The outbreak started to take hold in June to August 2014 in the eastern districts of Kailahun and Kenema, but it then spread westwards towards and into the areas around the capital, Freetown, with the highest numbers being reported in Port Loko district and the Western Rural and Western Urban areas after September 2014. It took until December 2014 for the number of care facilities and beds to be significantly increased, and prior to that time most of the victims were cared for in their homes and communities. It can be assumed that very few special arrangements were made for safe disposal of Ebola-contaminated human wastes up until the end of 2014.

It is against this background that the Government of Sierra Leone (Ministry of Water Resources and Ministry of Health and Sanitation) took the initiative to develop two guidance documents for use at the numerous Ebola care facilities which were being established across the country in 2014 and 2015.The first of these (Ministry of Water Resources, 2015a) addressed the likelihood of pollution of water resources by Ebola-contaminated wastes. The second (Ministry of Health and Sanitation, 2015) provided guidance on waste management at Ebola care facilities. These were being developed from the latter part of 2014 and into early 2015, and field-tested in early 2015. This paper discusses some of the issues which had to be considered and balanced in the preparation of those documents.

Once establishment of Ebola care facilities began in earnest towards the end of 2014, these took various forms, ranging from a few highly sophisticated structures such as that set up by UK forces in Kerry Town, to more numerous, remote and fairly basic community care centres in the smaller centres of population outside of the capital.

WASH issues at Ebola care facilities are threefold: first, the care facilities required significant quantities of water, especially for hygiene purposes. Relatively high volumes of water were needed for cleaning and washing down areas, and disinfecting personal protective equipment (PPE). This had implications for surface runoff and contamination, as construction of adequate drainage and soak-away systems was a real challenge in community care centres. Furthermore, a large proportion of existing wells and boreholes in Sierra Leone are known to be seasonal, so the availability of water could not be taken for granted.

The second issue is the subject of this paper: the large quantities of contaminated and potentially contaminated liquid and solid wastes produced at Ebola care facilities, all of which needed safe handling, containment, and management.

The third matter is the link between the first two. It appears that medical organizations often requested wells and water points to be sited within the care facility green zone, but this unfortunately placed them at a close proximity to the care facilities' latrine pits. This suggested that the potential for waterborne transmission may have been overlooked. In one case the water point is sited 5m from the wash-down area in the red zone, with drainage running directly towards the water point. In another example, at a community care facility set up by an international agency in a primary school, the treatment zone was located only metres away from the well used by the school and community, which the former consumers then refused to use.

Box 1. Basic information and assumptions about Ebola used in the guidance documents

Where is the Ebola virus? The Ebola virus can live and multiply in various animals (fruit bats and primates) and in the human body. Wastes originating in infected human populations and the care facilities where they are treated contain the virus. These wastes include human excreta and other body fluids; wastewater from washing of bodies, bed sheets and protective equipment; solid waste (including clinical waste); and corpses (WHO, 2014a).

Transmission. The Ebola virus is thought to be transmitted from fruit bats or primates to humans. Once in the human population, secondary human-to-human transmission occurs through direct contact with the blood, secretions, organs or other body fluids of infected persons. The risk of transmission is high for those caring for the sick, and for those handling bodies at funerals (WHO, 2014b).

Environmental contamination. Given Sierra Leone's wet climate (more than 2500mm of rain falling in the period April to November, with a peak in August, Ministry of Water Resources, 2015d), its very low coverage of improved sanitation (JMP, 2014), and the likelihood that not all those infected are admitted to care facilities, it should be assumed that the virus (along with faecal pollutants) is being released into the general environment. It may reach soil, surface water courses and groundwater. However, once there, its survival time is expected to be short (CDC, 2015).

Safe containment of contaminated waste below ground. If wastes containing the Ebola virus are contained in pits, the virus will survive there for a relatively short time (CDC, 2015). If it reaches the water table it will move with the groundwater flow, but such flow is very slow (Lawrence et al., 2001) and this gives time for the virus to die before it has travelled far. The best precaution that can be taken to prevent the Ebola virus entering drinking water supplies is to contain all contaminated wastes below ground (preferably well above the water table), while burning solid wastes, and avoid any subsequent excavation (e.g. de-sludging) of those pits. It is also important to avoid pits becoming flooded in the rainy season, as the consequent overflow of contaminated water will pollute surrounding soils and surface water courses. This applies both within Ebola care facility compounds and in villages and towns where Ebola victims are still present in the community.

It is highly unlikely that anyone will become infected via drinking water. The risk of contracting Ebola via a waterborne route is very small indeed. No case has been identified, in the current outbreak or any other, in which ingestion of Ebola-contaminated water has led to infection (CDC, 2015).

This guidance is about risk minimization. The guidance in this document is precautionary and the instructions presented here should not cause alarm. The best way of reducing the risk of water resources becoming contaminated with the Ebola virus is through good sanitation, waste management, and hygiene practice. These have many other benefits too.

Common basis

Both documents started from the then known and assumed information about the Ebola virus, its origin, its transmission and its survival. This information is well documented by the World Health Organisation (WHO, 2014b) and the US Centers for Disease Control (CDC, 2015). Box 1 provides a summary of this information, as used in the introduction to the two guidance documents.

Issues raised by the existing knowledge and the country context

A number of issues arise from the information in Box 1 and the context of Sierra Leone.

1. **Low risk, serious consequences**. No documented case of waterborne transmission of Ebola has been recorded. However, in very few specific cases is the actual route of transmission known with any certainty. Waterborne transmission may be unlikely, but were it to happen, its consequences would be very serious. Fatality rates due to Ebola are very high (57–60 per cent in the West African outbreak, WHO, 2015a) and those who recover from Ebola are subject to further medical complications and social stigma. By early 2015 there was already some anecdotal evidence that water users may have started to refuse to consume groundwater which they perceived might be contaminated with the Ebola virus.
2. **Survival and movement of the virus**. Outside the human body the Ebola virus is thought to survive for relatively short periods. However, survival for even a few days in a pit latrine, solid waste pit, soak-pit or grave would allow the virus to contaminate local groundwater in adverse conditions (e.g. shallow water table or rapid flow paths in the sub-surface). Sierra Leone experiences shallow water tables at the peak of the rains in August–September, and much of the country is underlain by crystalline (fractured) Basement Complex geology with a heterogeneous weathered zone containing many opportunities for rapid sub-surface flow. A review of the survival of the Ebola virus outside the human body (Bibby et al., 2015) drew this conclusion: '… while environmental exposure is not the dominant exposure route, available data suggest that it is imprudent to dismiss the potential of environmental transmission without further evidence. A significant research effort, including environmental persistence studies and microbial risk assessment, is necessary to inform the safe handling and disposal of Ebola virus contaminated waste, especially liquid waste in the wastewater collection and treatment system.'
3. **National context**. Sierra Leone has no functioning sewage treatment facilities, low levels of improved water supply and extremely

low levels of safe sanitation coverage (JMP, 2014), very basic solid waste management practices, weak public sector institutions and limited financial and human resources. It can safely be assumed that the ground surface and shallow soil are heavily contaminated with human and animal disease pathogens, especially in densely populated settlements, and the recent Ebola outbreak is likely to have added another virus, albeit a short-lived one, to the contamination load. The possibilities for safe management and containment of human and solid wastes (including clinical waste) in Sierra Leone are very limited. The majority of the population relies for their domestic water supply on water resources which are highly likely to be contaminated with human wastes and disease pathogens (Bain et al., 2014).
4. **Drafting guidance**. In the drafting of guidance, care needs to be taken (a) to recognize risk while not unnecessarily alarming the public, and (b) being very pragmatic while not restricting the management possibilities which may be achievable, even if higher standards can only be reached in a small minority of care facilities. Communicating uncertain science in simple prescriptive guidance is especially challenging.

Key aspects of Sierra Leone's climate and hydrogeology

Sierra Leone is a wet country, with a rainy season extending from April to November. National average annual rainfall is about 2,500mm, with values ranging from below 2,000mm in the north-east to over 4,000mm in the Freetown area (Ministry of Water Resources, 2015d).

About 80% of Sierra Leone is underlain by Basement Complex granites and other hard crystalline rocks, with an overlying clay-rich weathered zone. In addition there are significant areas of unconsolidated sediments near the coast, and a band of consolidated sedimentary rocks running south-east to north-west through the centre of the country (Ministry of Water Resources, 2015d).

Groundwater levels respond rapidly to the onset of rainfall (Ministry of Water Resources, 2015d), rising to within a few metres of the ground surface by mid-August, and then receding rapidly once the rate of recharge starts to reduce below the rate of natural discharge. The seasonal range of groundwater levels (dry season to rainy season) varies from less than 2m to about 8m.

The limited evidence suggests that (a) the shallow aquifers are recharged largely via rapid (vertical) flow paths during the rainy season, (b) natural outflow of groundwater to valleys is via rapid (sub-horizontal) flow routes, (c) groundwater levels are within a few metres of the ground surface for at least four months of the year, only receding to depths of greater than five metres in the dry season, and probably never in the lowland areas (Ministry of Water Resources, 2015d).

As a consequence, Sierra Leone's shallow aquifers may be especially vulnerable to groundwater pollution via diffuse (widespread) rapid vertical flow, and the seasonally shallow water tables may mean that relying on the unsaturated zone to attenuate pollution is unrealistic (Lapworth et al., 2015).

Key aspects of the guidance

The main assumptions and recommendations set out in the guidance documents were as follows:

1. **Wastes generated**. Ebola-contaminated liquid and solid wastes are generated in significant quantities within Ebola care facilities. There is a long list of such wastes, but they include body fluids (faeces, urine, blood, vomit), greywater (from washing, laundry and washdown of personal protective equipment, (PPE), used and damaged PPE, clinical waste and general organic and inorganic solid wastes.

2. **Waste containment**. As the equipment, resources and skills for waste management are very limited in Sierra Leone, all wastes generated within Ebola care facilities should be safely contained in pits of various kinds on-site. These include latrine pits, soak-pits, solid waste burial pits and sharps pits. It is highly unlikely that any of these would be lined pits. In the case of relatively dry solid waste, burning prior to burial is the preferred option. Given the lack of off-site waste treatment facilities in Sierra Leone, no contaminated or potentially contaminated waste should leave the site of the Ebola care facility.

3. **Burial of the dead**. While burials during 2014 mostly took place in the communities where the victims died, it was likely that, as care facilities became established from December 2014 onwards, an increasing number of burials took place near to those care facilities. The continuing risk to groundwater posed by burial sites and cemeteries is unknown.

4. **Groundwater pollution**. At the height of the outbreak it was highly likely that the virus would reach the water table, at least in the rainy season, and runoff from care facility sites at the peak of the rains means that surrounding soils and surface waters would also be contaminated. This pollution would persist for as long as the virus can survive, or for the duration of continuing inputs of Ebola-contaminated water, whichever is longer.

5. **Protection of water resources**. Protection of the surface waters and groundwaters which communities near to Ebola care facilities use for domestic supplies must rely on a sufficient vertical or horizontal separation distance between the care facility and the water point. Existing generic guidance on horizontal separation of pit latrines from wells (typically 15–50m, Graham and Polizzotto, 2013) is broadly applicable, as long as generalized contamination of the

environment can be minimized. The approach taken by Lawrence et al. (2001) may be too complex to apply in the Ebola outbreak, as it requires too much hard-to-gather data. Lapworth et al. (2015) concluded that vertical separation may present a better option, favouring properly constructed boreholes over shallow hand-dug wells for water supply.

Conclusions

The design of guidance on all aspects of the management of the Ebola crisis was challenging for at least these four reasons:

1. Ebola virus disease was only identified in 1976; there were 24 documented outbreaks prior to the West African crisis. Knowledge of the virus, especially its potential survival time outside the human body (in soil, water, waste and corpses), and of its exact mode of transmission is very limited.
2. If understanding of the actual risks to the public (for example from wastes and water pollution) is limited, public perception of risk, and how to manage it, are even less well understood.
3. Our ignorance of the disease and public understanding of the disease is matched by our limited knowledge of the natural environment – the properties and behaviour of the soil and sub-surface under the prevailing climatic conditions – in which water and wastes have to be managed.
4. The limited experience, resources, and capacity of national institutions in managing wastes, minimizing pollution, and protecting water resources restricts what is possible.

Nevertheless, pragmatic guidance had to be drafted, and it needed to be designed in such a way as to be achievable. The two guidance documents referred to in this paper attempted to be both pragmatic and useable. They are available from the Government of Sierra Leone.

End note

By March 2015 case numbers had dropped significantly in all three of the affected countries. The United Nations was expressing its confidence that the outbreak would be at an end by July–August 2015 (BBC, 2015). The World Health Organisation and others were starting to plan for decommissioning of Ebola Care Facilities (Day, S., pers. comm.). Draft guidance on this matter was mostly focused on minimization of the risk of the virus persisting in the environment. The important issue of public perception of risk – 'Is it safe to drink this water?' 'Is it safe to re-occupy school buildings which were used to care for Ebola victims?' 'What risks still persist from buried wastes and burial sites for the dead?' – has not yet been fully addressed. Careful sensitization and communication of risk to and with the public will be needed. Meanwhile two persistent unknowns remain. First, the ability of the virus to survive in soil, water, pit latrine contents and burial sites; and second, the risk posed by such possible survival to human beings. Before the next outbreak it will be important that the science has progressed on these matters.

About the authors

Richard C. Carter is a Consultant, Richard Carter and Associates Ltd, richard@richard-carter.org. **J. Peter Dumble** is a Consultant, Peter Dumble Hydrogeology, peter.dumble@PDHydrogeology.com. **St John Day** is a Consultant, Adam Smith International, StJohn.Day@adamsmithinternational.com. **Michael Cowing** is a Consultant, mjcowing@icloud.com

References

Bain, R., Cronk, R., Hossain, R., Bonjour, S., Onda, K., Wright, J., Yang, H., Slaymaker, T., Hunter, P., Prüss-Ustün, A., Bartram, J. (2014) 'Global assessment of exposure to faecal contamination through drinking water based on a systematic review'. *Tropical Medicine and International Health* 19 (8), pp917–927 <http://dx.doi.org/10.1111/tmi.12334>

BBC (2015) 'Ebola outbreak "over by August", UN suggests'. British Broadcasting Corporation News Site, 23rd March 2015 <http://www.bbc.co.uk/news/health-32009508>

Bibby, K., Casson, L. W., Stachler, E., and Haas, C. N. (2015) 'Ebola virus persistence in the environment: State of the knowledge and research needs', *Environmental Science and Technology Letters*, 2015, 2 (1) pp2–6. <http://dx.doi.org/10.1021/ez5003715> [last visited 19th January 2015].

CDC (2015) *Ebola (Ebola virus disease)*, <http://www.cdc.gov/vhf/ebola/> [last visited 14th January 2015].

Graham J. P. and Polizzotto (2013) 'Pit latrines and their impacts on groundwater quality: A systematic review', *Environmental Health Perspectives*, 121(5) pp 521–30, May 2013.

JMP (2014) *Progress on drinking water and sanitation, 2014 update*. World Health Organisation and UNICEF, <http://www.wssinfo.org/fileadmin/user_upload/resources/JMP_report_2014_webEng.pdf> [last visited 14th January 2015]

Lapworth, D. J., Carter, R. C., Pedley, S., MacDonald, A. M. (2015) 'Threats to groundwater supplies from contamination in Sierra Leone, with special reference to Ebola care facilities', British Geological Survey Open Report OR/15/009.

Lawrence, A. R., Macdonald, D. M. J., Howard, A. G., Barrett, M. H., Pedley, S., Ahmed, K. M., Nalubega, M. (2001) *Guidelines for assessing the risk to groundwater from on-site sanitation*. British Geological Survey, <http://www.bgs.ac.uk/downloads/search.cfm?SEARCH_TXT=argoss> [last visited 16th January 2015].

Ministry of Health and Sanitation (2015) *Waste management at Ebola care facilities. Part 1: Guidance note; part 2 Supplement*, Freetown, Government of Sierra Leone.

Ministry of Water Resources (2015a) *Protection of water resources from wastes at and around Ebola care facilities,* Freetown, Government of Sierra Leone.

Ministry of Water Resources (2015b) *Strategy for Water Security Planning,* Volume 1 of a three-volume set, Freetown, Government of Sierra Leone.

Ministry of Water Resources (2015c) *Water Resources Monitoring in Sierra Leone,* Volume 2 of a three-volume set, Freetown, Government of Sierra Leone.

Ministry of Water Resources (2015d) *Data and Hydrological Understanding in Sierra Leone,* Volume 3 of a three-volume set, Freetown, Government of Sierra Leone.

Visser, M. (2005) 'Ebola response in the Republic of Congo', *Waterlines* 23(3) 22–24.

WHO (2014a) *Ebola virus disease.* Fact sheet N°103, <http://www.who.int/mediacentre/factsheets/fs103/en/> [last visited 31 March 2015]

WHO (2014b) *Frequently asked questions on Ebola virus disease.* Updated August 2014. <http://www.who.int/csr/disease/ebola/faq-ebola/en/> [last visited 14th January 2015]

WHO (2015) *Global Alert and Response, Ebola Situation Report,* <http://www.who.int/csr/disease/ebola/situation-reports/en/> [last visited 14th January 2015].

CHAPTER 5
Menstrual hygiene management in humanitarian emergencies: gaps and recommendations

Marni Sommer

Abstract

Over the last 15 years there has been increasing attention to adolescent girls' and women's menstrual hygiene management (MHM) needs in humanitarian response contexts. A growing number of donors, non-governmental organizations, and governments are calling attention to the importance of addressing girls' and women's MHM-related needs in post-disaster and post-conflict settings. However, consensus on the most effective and culturally appropriate responses to provide for girls and women remains insufficiently documented for widespread sharing of lessons learned. This chapter is an effort to begin to document the recommendations of key multi-disciplinary experts working in humanitarian response on effective approaches to MHM in emergency contexts, along with a summarizing of the existing literature, and the identification of remaining gaps in MHM practice, research and policy in humanitarian contexts.

Keywords: menstrual hygiene management, humanitarian emergencies, adolescent girls, women

Over the last 15 years, there has been increasing attention within the global humanitarian emergency response community to addressing the menstrual hygiene management (MHM) needs of adolescent girls and women in post-conflict and post-disaster settings. MHM refers to the spectrum of interventions deemed necessary and appropriate to assure adolescent girls and women in various contexts can privately and safely manage their monthly menstrual flow. Although the global relief and development communities do not yet have an agreed definition of MHM per se, there is sufficient consensus to suggest that an MHM approach is multi-faceted, and includes adequate numbers of safe and private latrines (including separate latrines for girls and women with locks inside the doors); easily accessible water (ideally inside a latrine facility); culturally appropriate sanitary materials (cloth, pad); socially and environmentally appropriate means of disposal of used sanitary materials (e.g. burning, burying), or private washing/drying for cloths; and pragmatic information on hygienic menstrual management for pubescent girls who are reaching menarche or newly menstruating. There is currently a movement in

http://dx.doi.org/10.3362/9781780448831.005

the development community, particularly among those conducting research and programmes relating to water, sanitation, and education, to explore how best to assure schools in low-income countries are girl friendly in their ability to enable girls (and female teachers) to successfully manage their monthly menses. A growing body of literature delineates the minimal but expanding literature on this topic (Sommer 2009; Scott et al., 2009; Oster and Thornton 2009; Sommer 2010; Mahon and Fernandes, 2010; McMahon et al., 2011). In contrast, and likely owing to the nature of emergency work which provides insufficient time and added complexity to research and publications by experts in the field, there is less available evidence on the relief community's response writ large to addressing adolescent girls' and women's MHM needs.

The unique nature of the humanitarian response arena, that of focusing on life-saving measures as the priority in the immediate aftermath or acute phase of a natural disaster or eruption of conflict, and then assessing the appropriate interventions for sustained responses in differing situations (short-term versus long-term disaster settings; protracted conflict; internally displaced persons (IDPs) versus refugees; camp versus urban setting) lends an additional layer of complexity to determining what an appropriate MHM response should include, and when and how and by whom such a response is enacted. These were the types of situational context which served as a backdrop as the content of the paper was investigated. Key questions guiding the review included what is a typical MHM response; who usually enacts the response; when is an MHM response deemed appropriate; from where do the funds come to support MHM; and what are perceived existing gaps within the knowledge of the field and expert recommendations for improvement.

Review process

The review included three components: first, a desktop review was conducted of the grey and peer-reviewed literature as identified through searches of PubMed and other databases, along with Google and additional search engines. Second, inquiries were sent via electronic communication to key organizations working in humanitarian response (bilateral donors, United Nations agencies, and non-governmental organizations) to identify key experts to contact for interviews and documents that might not be identifiable through an internet search. Questions were also posted on a sanitation/menstruation-related blog requesting information on MHM in emergency response (SuSanA forum). Third, interviews were conducted by phone or email (questionnaires were utilized) to gather additional insights and perspectives into current MHM responses in humanitarian emergencies. Over 75 experts were contacted, with in-depth information gathered from a smaller sample of ~ 30 experts working in water and sanitation, reproductive health, and related areas. The findings from the combined searches are presented here, although individuals' names are not listed as permission was not requested to quote them on behalf of their respective agencies. A complete list of the documents reviewed is included in the reference list (although not all reports of UNHCR sanitary distributions have been included). This review did not incorporate the small but growing body of literature on MHM in development contexts.

The history of integrating MHM into emergency response

The inclusion of attention to menstrual-related needs within a standard emergency response seems to have emerged after the 1994 Beijing platform in which attention was called to the reproductive rights and dignity of women. A more systematic effort to address MHM can be traced to a few specific documented efforts: 1) the United Nations High Commission for Refugees' (UNHCR) five commitments to refugee women delineated over a decade ago when providing sanitary materials to women became a noted priority for the agency (UNHCR, 2011a); 2) although a newer actor in the humanitarian field, the United Nations Population Fund's (UNFPA) emphasis on the provision of 'dignity kits' to adolescent girls and women in humanitarian responses, which frequently include sanitary materials, soap and underwear depending on the local context; and 3) the ever-expanding inclusion of MHM (or mention of menstruation-related needs) in the Sphere Standards, which will be discussed below. Additional sources of historical inclusion of MHM as an important part of an emergency response can be found within selected non-governmental organizations' (NGOs) standard operations, such as Oxfam and the International Federation of the Red Cross and Red Crescent Societies (IFRC), although many NGOs' records of MHM efforts are contained within internal organization documents that are not publicly available for review. The history and range of different organizations' approaches to MHM, such as the distribution of hygiene kits and construction of private, safe latrines, is more extensive than can be captured in this one chapter. This is particularly the case given the minimal written reports that exist on MHM, and the differing contextual nature of past emergency responses which have varied depending on the type of emergency and its geographic, cultural, and economic setting.

Existing guidance documents on integrating MHM into emergency response

The existing guidance or guidelines on recommended approaches to addressing adolescent girls' and women's menstrual-related needs in emergency responses can be found in a range of sources. Although not all guidance documents are used by all sectors or organizations, the existing mentions of MHM are useful for delineating if and what additional guidance may be needed to assure MHM is appropriately incorporated in future emergency response.

The *Sphere Minimum Standards for Humanitarian Response*, now in its third edition, have included increasingly detailed mention of menstruation with each subsequent revision (Sphere 2000; 2004; 2011). The content on menstrual-related response is primarily located in the WASH section of the

Sphere Handbook, with suggestions made regarding privacy of latrines/toilets, provision of sanitary materials, and disposal of used sanitary materials. The most recent *Sphere Handbook* edition (2011) recommends consultation with local women about their preferred menstrual sanitary materials (with one cloth recommended per woman); the promotion of women's involvement in water supply and sanitation approaches; the provision of underwear and a washing basin as additional items; the need for basins and laundry areas for women (for washing of sanitary materials and underwear); the availability of disposal mechanisms for used sanitary materials; and attention to schoolgirls' menstrual-related needs. The Handbook does not provide details on how to conduct the consultations with adolescent girls and women as this may fall beyond its purview as standards (versus guidelines). It also does not include recommendations regarding the placement of water inside latrines/toilets for privacy of washing menstrual-related stains and cloths.

The Inter-Agency Working Group on Reproductive Health in Crises (IAWG), the *Inter-agency Field Manual on Reproductive Health in Humanitarian Settings* (2010), and the guidance within the Minimal Initial Services Package (MISP) distance learning module focuses on priority reproductive health services with additional guidance on menstrual-related responses, such as the provision of basic hygiene kits for all women and girls, ordered locally, and a three month supply of sanitary materials, underwear, soap, and towels (MISP, 2007). The UNFPA *Adolescent Sexual and Reproductive Health Toolkit for Humanitarian Settings* mentions a minimum standard as the provision of sanitary materials to adolescent girls, and as part of a comprehensive response, the provision of puberty education for 10–14 year olds (with the suggestion that such information would address menstrual management) (UNFPA, 2009). The report emphasizes the need to consult with adolescent girls on any planned intervention. Another useful document that incorporates questions about cultural beliefs pertaining to menstrual management into its assessment guidance is the *Inter-Agency Standing Committee Gender Handbook in Humanitarian Action* (IASC, 2006).

From the education emergency response community, an extensive discussion of how to respond to adolescent schoolgirls' and women teachers' menstrual-related needs is found in a report by the Inter-Agency Network for Education in Emergencies (INEE) Gender Task Team (2006) using the INEE Minimum Standards as a framework for a tool entitled *Gender Responsive School Sanitation, Health and Hygiene*. The guidance includes assuring appropriate solid waste disposal, adequate water, separate toilets, and provision of sanitary materials for schoolgirls and female teachers. Emphasis is placed on the possibility that girls and teachers may miss school if these conditions are not met. The guidance document also suggests that existing curricula may be inadequate for providing girls with the pragmatic menstrual hygiene information they need, and that families in crisis situations may lack time to teach girls about such needs. A multi-disciplinary response is recommended, one that incorporates distribution of non-food items (NFIs), education, water, sanitation, and health.

Additional guidance is included in UN and NGO documents, such as UNHCR's *Handbook for the Protection of Women and Girls* (2008) which highlights the need for attention to the asylum seeker's need for sanitary materials, available disposal, and bathing facilities; and emphasizes the potential negative outcomes of not providing such services, including the potential for girls' school attendance to decrease, and for girls to exchange sex for money in order to afford sanitary pads. Case study examples are included, such as Nike Foundation's support for private and separate latrines for schoolgirls in Kenya (UNHCR, 2008). A recent UNHCR survey of 88 country offices that explored the need to update UNHCR's guidance and support for the inclusion of MHM-related interventions includes mention of the UNHCR standard response of the provision of pads/cloth, underwear, and soap, with reports from the field suggesting girls and women are in need of a separate basin for washing of menstrual-related cloths/underwear for hygienic and cultural reasons, such as taboos that prevent washing of such materials in the family's primary wash basin. Obstacles identified to the inclusion of MHM (primarily the provision of sanitary materials) in country experiences will be incorporated into the section below (UNCHR, 2011).

The guidance documents from most organizations operating in emergencies, such as the International Committee of the Red Cross (ICRC), Oxfam, CARE, the Office of Foreign Disaster Assistance (OFDA), UNHCR, and others, are primarily internal. Useful information was, however, gleaned from UNHCR, UNFPA, OFDA, and those NGOs more actively exploring whether their current MHM-related responses are as effective as they should be, and how they might be revised (UNHCR, 2011c; Abbott et al., 2011). One example is IFRC, which has traditionally distributed hygiene kits during the acute phase of disaster emergencies and then monitored and revised as needed in the subsequent phases of the disasters. Based on selected experiences where the agency felt the incorrect sanitary material was provided, such as sanitary pads to women who were unfamiliar and uncomfortable with their usage, the WASH group is proposing a revised response where only soap and water storage are distributed until the WASH staff engages in dialogue with the beneficiaries about their preferred materials (IFRC, 2011). The effort would aim to ensure WASH staff are engaged in both the development of the kit through consultations with beneficiaries, and also training in the use and promotion of the kits. A positive impact would be the distribution of more appropriate materials and hence increased uptake and use, while a negative potential impact might be a multiple week delay in the provision of any sanitary materials to adolescent girls and women given the time needed to procure and receive supplies. An alternative approach is used by NGOs such as Oxfam, which prefers to distribute materials immediately if the need is apparent (e.g. frequently they distribute a piece of cloth such as kanga or sari to free up the use of women's other cloths), with subsequent monitoring to revise errors in the MHM response. The guidance provided to staff of any NGO may also be influenced by the type of organization it is and how it operates in the field, such as those international NGOs with permanent staff based in countries or regions when emergencies occur or who fly in technical experts to respond, versus, for example, the IFRC, which operates through its 187 national societies, which take the lead in an emergency and can provide important cultural inputs, in collaboration with an extensive volunteer pool of technical experts who may have less expertise on an issue such as MHM (although trainings are conducted to try to address such gaps).

Assessment tools

There are numerous assessment tools that are used in the field, including initial rapid assessments, baseline assessments for the post-acute phase, the Participatory Hygiene and Sanitation Transformation Process (PHAST), Minimum Initial Service Package (MISP), and donor, UN, or NGO assessment tools. While there were differing opinions as to when and how questions on MHM should be incorporated into tools, there was a clear consensus that additional guidance was needed. Such guidance might include minimal questions for inclusion early in the emergency life-saving phase, with more detailed guidance provided for longer-term response situations in which field teams would utilize participatory methodologies to explore adolescent girls' and women's menstrual-related needs and preferences given the frequently taboo and secretive nature of the topic. The importance of using participatory and more empowering methodologies is described in a useful case study describing the use of PHAST after the Pakistan 2005 earthquake (IFRC, 2006). Suggestions were also made for preplanning guidance, with one possibility being a 'mapping' of menstrual practices (cultural beliefs around materials, disposal, sanitation) used by girls and women in countries around the world so MHM supplies and related responses could be appropriately pre-positioned in regions. The author recently conducted a global review of menstrual practices which might prove a useful starting place for such a mapping, although the literature was scant (Sommer, 2011). Another suggestion was to pre-prepare and pre-position MHM promotion materials for staff, teachers, and adolescent girls in local languages, much as the WASH field has done for other hygiene-related topics.

The existing guidance and assessment tools provide insight into the various sectors who traditionally respond to MHM-related needs, ranging from the WASH (water, sanitation, and hygiene) sector to reproductive health, or education. From the range of interviews conducted, there appears to be a predominance of MHM elements noted in relation to WASH responses in emergencies, particularly as relates to the hygiene promotion sphere, although the reproductive health sector has served an important role in the inclusion of hygiene kits (e.g. sanitary materials). The various logistics of the responses will be further discussed below; however it seems important that future revisions of guidance and assessment tools clearly delineate which sectors will be responsible for which components of

MHM, including coordination with other relevant sectors, in order to minimize overlap and maximize response effectiveness.

The literature on integrating MHM into emergency response

Much of the existing minimal literature on MHM in emergency responses can be found in a search of the grey literature or through contacting individual experts as mentioned above at organizations engaged in emergency post-disaster and post-conflict response. The search of the peer-reviewed literature did not identify any specific articles focused on MHM responses in emergencies (with one exception on Pakistan described below), although mention of the need to better address this topic was found in a small selection of articles focused on MHM in development contexts. Both organization reports and case study examples presented at various conferences proved to be useful sources of field experts' views on possible responses. A repeated example mentioned by experts was MHM-related responses to different emergencies in Pakistan over the last six years, with discussion of the confusion that arose among men and women when disposable sanitary pads were distributed (e.g. men utilized the pads for other purposes not recognizing they were menstrual sanitary materials), and agencies' efforts to improve their MHM responses in subsequent Pakistan emergencies. The latter included a very useful article and Water, Development and Engineering Centre (WEDC) conference briefing paper delineating the effort to build appropriate sanitation and water facilities for adolescent girls and women, and the input from beneficiaries that was crucial to the incorporation of private menstrual material washing and drying spaces. The latter included the need for entry into the facilities to be hidden from the opposite sex (Nawaz et al., 2006, 2010). Such examples highlight the critical need for contextualization of an MHM response both in terms of the local cultural and geographic setting, and the type and timeline of the selected emergency. Another useful WEDC briefing paper addressed the MHM challenges facing women in northern Ugandan IDP camps, highlighting the insufficient materials, privacy, sanitation, and bathing facilities experienced by women, and the lack of MHM guidance for girls. The paper discusses the subsequent UNICEF-supported response to address MHM challenges in collaboration with IDP women (Bwengye-Kahororo and Twanza, 2005). There is a great need for additional case study examples to be provided to enhance the literature on possible approaches to addressing MHM in a sensitive and effective manner. Although numerous brief news or organizational reports exist online mentioning the distribution of sanitary materials in humanitarian scenarios ranging from Uganda to Yemen to Aceh, insufficient detail is included to allow for much learning. As will also be discussed below, a key question emerging from the document review and interviews was the need for improved evaluation and follow up of existing MHM responses, and publications highlighting relevant findings.

In building the MHM in emergency response literature in the coming years, attention should also be paid to where such publications are located, given the likelihood that experts within the WASH sector will be focused on water- and sanitation-related articles, while experts in the reproductive health and education sectors may focus on articles published within their respective fields. Conflict- or disaster-specific journals or databases would also be a good place for experts to learn about the different sector responses, and case study examples that become available.

Viewpoints on integrating MHM into emergency response

The current status of the field of MHM in humanitarian emergency responses that emerged from the review seemed to be one that is increasingly systematic but not yet sufficiently so, and one that is in need of additional guidance, evaluation, and even clarity of underlying purpose and aims across the emergency response field. The more effective MHM-related responses appeared to be dependent on the organization, experience, and commitment level in relation to MHM of the staff involved (as with so many programmatic responses). Improvement of the larger field of those engaging (or not yet engaging) in MHM responses, it was recommended, would be most effectively strengthened if improved guidance on assessment and response in various contexts, including clarifying of sector roles and responsibilities, and training on the issue are provided in the future. More specific thematic areas that emerged as key aspects of current (and future) MHM response in emergencies will be discussed one by one below. The overall consensus appeared to be that MHM was not yet sufficiently incorporated as standard practice in emergencies, or integrated in a systematic way, with current staff trainings (WASH, reproductive health, education), which have inadequate MHM content.

What does MHM response typically include?

The typical MHM response includes all or some of the following components: the provision of sanitary materials (cloth and/or disposable pads), soap, and possibly related items (e.g. underwear, basin) through the distribution of hygiene promotion kits; and the construction of safe and private water and sanitation facilities (with the latter also addressing the need for privacy, water, and space for laundering and bathing). The distribution of hygiene kits is often a one-time distribution during the acute phase of the emergency or immediately thereafter, with less attention to menstrual sanitary material needs afterwards. The expectation and hope amongst many emergency staff is that after the one-time distribution, adolescent girls and women will be able to return to their usual menstrual practices (whether perceived as hygienic or not by the emergency staff), with minimal follow up to assess if adolescent girls and women in protracted conflicts or long-term disaster settings feel adequately supported during menses.

The construction of appropriate water, sanitation, bathing, and laundering facilities is a critical component of a typical MHM response, although one that to date may have inadequately incorporated adolescent girls' and women's specific preferences and needs. Decisions over what gets constructed and how will obviously depend on the nature of the emergency and the priority aim of life-saving interventions and the prevention of infectious disease. However subsequent to assuring the latter, organizations can be creative, such as the Pakistan case study example in which menstrual washing and drying spaces were devised (and amended as needed), along with the findings of why women did or did not choose to use the facilities published to provide insights for future emergency responses. Assuring such facilities are safe and private is essential, with cultural appropriateness an ideal. For example, an Oxfam intervention with women in the DRC that was aimed at assuring appropriate disposal of used menstrual materials revealed that burning menstrual blood was taboo. So a discussion was commenced with local women to devise an appropriate alternative approach, which resulted in the burying of used menstrual materials in a safe manner.

The content of the hygiene promotion kits differs by agency or organization distributing or procuring the items; UNFPA's dignity kits are frequently composed of items procured locally, while IFRC as mentioned, will be re-examining whether kits should be pre-positioned and distributed prior to consultation with beneficiaries. Many organizations, such as Oxfam and ICRC, pre-position kits in selected regions, distribute what is contained during the acute phase (if needed) and then monitor and assess if the response is appropriate or needs amending. Decisions on what to contain in the pre-positioned kits are usually made in consultation with local country staff more familiar with local cultural menstrual practices. Many organizations provide sanitary materials and soap, but not underwear (which may render the materials inadequate if the girls and women are unable to use them); while other organizations distribute cloth (given its frequent cultural acceptability) but do not account for the need for girls and women to wash and dry the materials privately and with adequate water and soap. In contexts of extreme drought, for example, the increased need for water during monthly menses may not be adequately accounted for by all emergency actors. Organizations also differ by whether they purchase items for the hygiene kits locally or procure internationally, although the latter decision is frequently made on a case-by-case basis depending on what the local market contains, and the economics around purchasing the maximum materials with the funding available. One creative example from a protracted conflict is that of Uganda where UNHCR has engaged in a partnership with Makerere University and GTZ, employing refugee women to produce environmentally friendly disposal pads made of papyrus leaves (Maka pads). While some reports suggest Maka pads are useful but not sufficient for girls' and women's heaviest menstrual flow days, this is still a good example of a locally based solution. Other examples include the re-useable AfriPads being produced in Uganda and the pads made by women's groups in the camps in Dadaab. Another approach is the one time partnership between UNHCR and Proctor & Gamble (P&G), in which the latter provided disposable sanitary pads en masse to the organization. This collaboration was deemed effective with P&G covering the costs of transporting the pads.

The discussion of the typical MHM response leads to a consideration of differing but overlapping perspectives that emerged during the review about the justification for addressing MHM in emergencies, an issue which would be useful to clarify and gain consensus on in the future. One perspective is that the inclusion of MHM serves the primary role of meeting adolescent girls' and women's health and hygiene needs, and preventing the possibility of infection if not hygienically managed (although the latter is less frequently mentioned). A second perspective perceives attention to MHM as an issue of protection, emphasizing the dangers (primarily sexually related) existing for adolescent girls and women who are not sufficiently provided with private and safe facilities, and an adequate supply of sanitary materials. The third perspective perceives the role of an MHM response as a life-saving measure (and hence equates it with other acute phase interventions) given the need for adolescent girls and women to join the long queues for water or food distributions, and other challenges of providing essential needs for their families in emergency contexts, and the difficulties of doing so if lacking adequate sanitary materials and facilities. The fourth perspective perceives the MHM response (and particularly the provision of kits) as an issue of dignity, and one that is crucial for girls and women to feel empowered to engage in survival and other daily activities in an emergency context. Lastly, the fifth is that of the education perspective, and the need for adolescent girls and female teachers to participate in education in emergency contexts, and hence the need for appropriate MHM responses in the school setting. While all of these perspectives overlap to some degree, clarification amongst emergency experts on the overall rationale for incorporating MHM into emergency response as an essential component would prove useful.

Who conducts MHM response (assessment, intervention, evaluation)?

There are a variety of actors engaged in the MHM response in post-conflict and post-disaster contexts. There does not appear to be a total consensus on whose responsibility MHM ultimately is, particularly when related to the hygiene kits, with both WASH/hygiene promotion and reproductive health having a role in different past emergencies. In terms of assessment, individual organizations (NGOs, donors, UN) conduct their own assessments and particularly in the acute phase of a conflict, collaborate within sectors on the appropriate response. While the WASH sector usually takes responsibility for the construction of water and sanitation facilities, they may also be engaged in the procurement of non-food items (NFIs) which frequently include hygiene kits (although the content of the kits can as mentioned vary). The procurement of hygiene kits can differ, sometimes coming through a UN agency such as UNFPA or UNICEF, while in other contexts NGOs such as CARE and Oxfam will create their own kits either through their WASH or reproductive health point people. It is less clear who should focus on assessing the needs of schools in emergency settings to assure MHM-related interventions are incorporated to address girls' and female teachers' water and sanitation needs, along with the provision of sanitary materials and pragmatic menstrual management guidance for girls who are lacking information. This is likely a collaborative response between the WASH and education or protection sectors.

The issue of assessment also raises questions of how the assessment is conducted. Some organizations rely during the acute phase of the conflict on their local staff for menstrual-related information, as such staff may be more familiar with cultural practices relating to menstruation, while in later aspects of the emergency, such as during the early recovery period, staff (preferably female and frequently hygiene promotion workers) will conduct participatory assessments or a survey of adolescent girls' and women's needs. Understandably, there appears to be a trade-off between wanting to respond quickly and with urgency, and assuring that whatever the MHM response encompasses, it is culturally and socially appropriate so as not to prove useless and disempowering to girls and women. Many agencies emphasize the need for consultation with beneficiaries in their guidance materials, although additional and more explicit guidance on how to explore the issue of menses management was recommended. One recommendation included the use of visual aids on MHM for staff to use with beneficiaries, such as those utilized by UNICEF/Bangladesh or included in the WASH VAL (visual aids from WASH cluster). Surveys may be less effective for eliciting such information, while focus group discussions may take more time but more effectively gather sensitive information, a methodological trade-off that needs to be negotiated in each emergency context.

The monitoring and evaluation of MHM responses is an area deemed particularly lacking in past and current emergency responses. While some organizations conduct monitoring of interventions, such as the uptake and use of the facilities to assure they are being utilized by girls and women, multiple sources reported a significant gap in the field's understanding of feedback on how menstrual hygiene kits may or may not have met girls' and women's needs, and follow-up post-distribution of kits to ascertain ongoing needs. One example of challenges that can arise in the evaluations occurred in a remote province in Afghanistan where an NGO attempted to evaluate its WASH programme. The international consultant hired to conduct the evaluation (a woman) was not allowed to travel to the rural areas to meet with local women for security reasons, and the local women were not allowed to travel to the provincial capital for cultural reasons. An effort to hire a female translator to conduct a Skype session with the rural women proved equally problematic given that only one local woman in the province was known to be sufficiently educated to be able to translate, and she was not available. The consultant had to work with a male translator and a male in the rural area managing the technology, which prohibited any questions being asked about

MHM given the cultural context. Such examples are essential to incorporate into the literature so that others attempting to evaluate MHM-related projects can try to plan for such challenges in similar contexts.

The consensus appeared to be that while increasing numbers of organizations are incorporating MHM into their responses, the existing guidance is insufficient, and the various components of MHM are rarely all included, with kits provided in some settings, water and sanitation in others, and more infrequently, adequate bathing and laundering facilities. The provision of menses management guidance to girls is an even less mentioned topic, aside from the education and sexual and reproductive health sectors, although one example was the inclusion of a Tanzania puberty book (www.growandknow.org, 'publications' link) which was created for a development context and was recently shared during UNHCR-supported WASH trainings in sub-Saharan Africa, and incorporated into the associated UNHCR WASH training CD for various countries in East, the Horn of, and Central Africa.

When is MHM response appropriate during an emergency?

There were differing viewpoints on when MHM is most appropriate during an emergency response, although the conclusion appeared to be that immediate distribution of sanitary materials (hygiene kits) should be a priority, along with the construction of water and sanitation facilities (although these would be built regardless of MHM for disease prevention purposes). There was, as mentioned, some disagreement over the kit distribution approach, and the suggestion that local consultations with beneficiaries should occur before any sanitary materials are procured or distributed, even though this would slow the response likely by many weeks. In terms of consultation with beneficiaries (girls and women) over the adequacy of water, sanitation, laundering, and bathing facilities for MHM-related needs, it was less clear when in the scope of an emergency this is recommended, although these consultations appeared to occur during the early recovery phase of the emergency and less so in the acute phase. The nature of the rapid assessment questionnaire in most emergency contexts is one that needs to be short and focused on preventing disease outbreaks. Opinions on whether or not it would be appropriate to include questions on MHM into these rapid questionnaires varied, although consensus seemed to be that it might not be appropriate unless it meant adding only one targeted question. If a question were to be included, attention should be given to ensure it was asked in a sensitive way, and in adherence to local cultural norms and taboos.

The conclusion, although this is one of the issues that would best be debated and determined by experts leading the field of emergency response, is that an immediate standardized and systematic MHM response in terms of distribution of kits is preferred, with subsequent (and soon thereafter) monitoring and evaluation assuring the tailoring of the hygiene materials distributed and the water, sanitation, laundering, and bathing facilities constructed to girls and women's MHM-related needs. Emergency responders can best assess if it would be preferable to construct the facilities according to girls' and women's needs from the start, based on the size, context, and nature of the emergency.

Which beneficiaries are usually targeted for MHM response?

The primary focus of staff in terms of MHM-related assessment and intervention appeared to be primarily on women of reproductive age, with younger menstruating adolescent girls and older women with delayed menopause frequently overlooked. The more experienced organizations appear to make a stronger effort to separate out adolescent girls and women, with examples provided of decisions to distribute disposable pads to girls and cloth to women based on their stated preferences (including a report given of one occasion when older women who were given cloth became jealous of the girls' disposable pads).

One of the frequent challenges reported by those working in emergencies is those contexts in which multiple cultural groups, ages, and socioeconomic classes are all together, and the difficulty of identifying what the appropriate materials should be to distribute (along with the cost-effectiveness of responding to differing preferences). Other organizations reported examples of how when emergencies occur in urban settings, they are more likely to distribute disposable sanitary pads, while for emergencies in rural contexts, they are more likely to include cloths in the kits. Some organizations include both cloth and disposal pads in their kits, while other organizations first consult with local staff to assure they procure the appropriate colour and material for the cloth.

In terms of the distribution of kits, there was some consensus that overlap occurs, and agencies and organizations would do better to clarify their target beneficiaries both in terms of assessment, and in terms of distribution and evaluation (Abbott et al., 2011). Such targeting would also be important for gathering input with regard to the use of water and sanitation facilities, as adolescent girls may have responsibilities and preferences and face dangers going about their daily activities in an emergency setting that are different from those of older women. A priority emphasized by most organizations was the need to consult with adolescent girls and women in a sensitive and appropriate manner that will elicit the needed information. An excellent example was given by one interviewee who described the difference in gathering information on menstrual material preferences from a group of urban women who may be used to publicly purchasing disposable sanitary materials, compared with adolescent girls living in rural Sudan who may have never spoken out loud to anyone about their monthly menses and how they manage it.

Where does funding come from for MHM?

The availability of funding for integrating MHM into emergency responses appeared to be a significant issue, and partially related to the under-funded nature of the sanitation and reproductive health sectors in general. Other potential reasons for the funding challenges may be related to the fact that

MHM has to date been frequently overlooked by the emergency community; to the lack of a clear 'home' for MHM within the various emergency sectors; or because of a lack of clarity on how best to respond (and what to fund). Funds primarily come from UN agencies, bilateral donors such as OFDA, the private sector (such as P&G's donation of pads), and through organizations' own internal fundraising mechanisms (Dawn, 2008; P&G, 2010). A number of experts suggested that greater attention needs to be paid to educating the donor community about why MHM should be prioritized (and hence funded) in emergencies. Given UNHCR's inclusion of MHM in standard assistance packages, the UNHCR survey of their country offices was particularly revealing in highlighting that budgetary issues were a frequent reason why MHM was not incorporated (or did not have sustained inclusion) in their responses. In response, headquarters is determined to assure that in the future MHM is treated as a priority, essential component of country-level responses.

Why does MHM get overlooked?

There are numerous reasons why MHM may in the past, and still in the present, be overlooked in emergency response. Some of the reasons overlap with those of the development community which has also overlooked MHM until now, but other reasons are likely to be related to the unique nature of emergency response. First, as various experts suggested, the water and sanitation community was for a long time predominantly male, a group who may have unintentionally overlooked girls' and women's menstrual needs given their lack of personal experience with the challenges that monthly menses present. Second, and related, men (and women) may be uncomfortable discussing and asking about the issue of menstruation, particularly in different cultural contexts where the topic is particularly taboo. So this in turn may lead to its absence from the response plan. Third, those focused on the immediate life-saving needs of an acute emergency (e.g. disease prevention, emergency obstetric care) may from their training and orientation within the field of public health in emergencies, not consider MHM a relevant aspect of immediate need. This latter reason would bump up against the earlier discussion of the justifications for including an MHM response immediately, that of the perception that it may in fact be life-saving. Fourth, given the frequently taboo nature of the topic (even in industrialized countries) it is unlikely that adolescent girls and women will clamour for help regarding their MHM needs, in comparison with needs for shelter, food, and water, unless specifically approached and asked in a sensitive manner.

What are the unique aspects of responding to MHM?

In assessing and responding to adolescent girls' and women's menstrual management needs in a range of contexts, from rural Africa or Pakistan to urban Asia and Haiti, there is a need for the relevant actors within the emergency response community to understand the local menstrual beliefs and practices that may be relevant for an effective response. Numerous taboos and secrecy still exist around discussing menstruation and its management, with cultural beliefs particularly important for the materials that are used to manage it, the design of the water and sanitation facilities with regard to privacy, and the disposal of used materials. Most of these beliefs can be adequately assessed if sensitive approaches are used to engage adolescent girls and women, but it is important for staff to recognize that some girls and women, particularly in more rural contexts, may never have discussed the issue openly before (or even shared it with their mothers) (Sommer 2009; McMahon et al., 2011). Staff themselves may also be less comfortable addressing the MHM topic, and hence the suggestion that additional training and awareness raising occur.

Gaps in knowledge on MHM response in emergencies

As already mentioned, there are a number of gaps in the current knowledge on responding to MHM in emergency contexts, including the differing justifications for incorporating MHM. These gaps include the shortage of evaluations conducted on what has and has not worked in past emergencies, including more specifically the views of beneficiaries on the usefulness of the kits and materials distributed and what their ongoing needs may be in differing contexts (such as short- or long-term disasters and protracted conflicts); along with beneficiaries' views on the effectiveness (or not) of water, sanitation, laundering (including privacy for washing and drying of cloths), and bathing facilities constructed in various emergency settings. There exists insufficient information on why MHM has not been fully integrated to date as a standard part of an emergency response, including the barriers to doing so, and how best to overcome such barriers to assure that adolescent girls' and women's MHM-related needs are effectively met in a timely manner. Lastly, and related to all of the above-mentioned reasons, there is little documentation of NGOs' standard practices in terms of either assessing or responding to MHM in various types of emergency, potentially contributing to the current absence of a systematic MHM response based on documented experience and evaluation.

Recommendations for improving MHM response in emergencies

Numerous organizations reported a renewed or new commitment to better addressing MHM in emergency responses, citing the dedication of their organizations' directors to assuring adolescent girls' and women's menstrual-related needs are adequately and effectively addressed. The challenge is translating this strong commitment into a more widespread commitment assuring MHM is systematically, sensitively, efficiently, and effectively incorporated into emergencies (broadly defined for various contexts and situations) as deemed most appropriate by those experts working day to day in the field. This necessitates flexibility in response depending on the context and emergency. Some key recommendations that emerged from this review of the existing documentation and expert opinion included the following: One, there should be a delineated systematic response to MHM with a clear assignment of roles that incorporates the multi-disciplinary components of an MHM response. Two, this systematic response should assure that a coordinated assessment and response is enacted by including the primary actors of relevance (e.g. shelter, WASH, reproductive health, education). Three, improved and more detailed guidance is needed on how best to assess, intervene, and evaluate MHM in emergencies, so those operating in fast-moving emergencies have clarity on how best to gather information and act on it. Four, emergency organizations should consider additional mechanisms for planning for MHM-related aspects of emergencies, such as the suggested mapping of countries' traditional practices and beliefs around preferred sanitary materials and appropriate mechanisms of disposal through local collaborators. Five, organizations or UN agencies might consider utilizing the existing Tanzania puberty book (with adaptations already occurring in additional African and Asian countries) or other existing books such as those available in India, Zimbabwe, Sierra Leone, and Afghanistan, in a format that could be quickly adapted and distributed in longer-term emergency contexts where numerous young girls approaching menarche can be found. Six, and lastly, adequate and clear funding streams must be identified for assuring all the MHM components are able to be incorporated into emergency responses when deemed appropriate.

Conclusion

In conclusion, there appears to be a strong and growing interest in better addressing adolescent girls' and women's MHM-related needs in humanitarian emergency contexts, paired with a lack of systematic guidance on how to most effectively respond. Much rich expertise abounds amongst the emergency response community, with seeming consensus on most of the priority gaps in information and the recommendations for an improved way forward. The aim of conducting this review was to provide an up-to-date, albeit brief, summary of the status of MHM responses in emergencies in an effort to assist those attempting to move the MHM agenda ahead in emergency contexts. While this review is not intended to be all encompassing, the input from the various experts working in the challenging emergency contexts of today's world provided extraordinarily helpful insights into the topic of MHM in humanitarian response.

Acknowledgements

My greatest appreciation and thanks go to two exceptional students who assisted with this review, Hannah Needleman and Rebecca Kruger. My additional great appreciation is extended to all the emergency experts who amidst their busy schedules took the time to respond to our many questions and provide their insights. Particular thanks are extended to Sarah House,

William Carter, Marion O'Reilly, Janet Meyers, Irene Van Horssen, Sandra Krause, Suzanne Ferron, Henia Dakkak, Trevor White, and Ashley Hernreich.

About the author

Marni Sommer (ms2778@columbia.edu) is Associate Professor of Sociomedical Sciences, Mailman School of Public Health, Columbia University.

References

Abbott, L., Bailey, B., Karasawa, Y., Louis, D., McNab, S., Patel, D., Lopez, C., Rani, R., Saba, C. and Vaval, L. (2011) *Evaluation of UNFPA's Provision of Dignity Kits in Humanitarian and Post-crisis Settings*, SIPA, New York.

Bharadwaj, S. and Patkar, A. (2004) *Menstrual Hygiene and Management in Developing Countries: Taking Stock* [website] http://www.mum.org/menhydev.htm [accessed 24 August 2011].

Bwengye-Kahororo, E. and Twanza, E. (2005) 'Promoting women's hygiene in emergency situations', briefing paper submitted to *31st WEDC International Conference*, Kampala, Uganda.

Dawn, C. (2008) *Corporate Gift Highlights Sanitation Problems Faced by Female Refugees* [website], UNHCR http://www.unhcr.org/4815db792.html [accessed 1 August 2011].

Fleischman, J. (2011) *Re-usable Sanitary Pads Helping Keep Girls in School, The Commission on Smart Global Health Policy*, Center for Strategic and International Studies, Washington, DC.

Group URD and Academie de l'Eau (2009) *Water and Sanitation in Emergency and Post-crisis Contexts*, Group URD, Plaisians, France.

Harris, S. (1999) 'Homogenising humanitarian assistance to IDP communities (a cautionary note from Sri Lanka)', *Forced Migration Review* 4: 19-21.

Harris, S. (2000) 'Listening to the displaced: Analysis, accountability and advocacy in action', *Forced Migration Review* 8: 20-21.

IFRC (2006) *South Asia Earthquake – Pakistan: Ensuring Gender Equity and Community Participation in the WatSan Programme*, IFRC, Geneva.

IFRC (2011) 'WatSan and Health NFI's Overview and Guidelines', unpublished draft concept note, IFRC, Geneva.

INEE (2006) *Gender Responsive School Sanitation, Health and Hygiene* [website], INEE http://toolkit.ineesite.org/resources/ineecms/uploads/1042/Gender_Strategies_in_Emergencies.PDF [accessed 21 April 2015].

Integrated Regional Support Program (2011) *Menstrual Hygiene Kits Distribution* [website], http://irsp.org.pk/2011/01/menstrual-hygiene-kits-distribution/ [accessed 13 December 2011].

IASC (Inter-Agency Standing Committee) (2006) *Gender Handbook in Humanitarian Action* http://www.humanitarianinfo.org/iasc/pageloader.aspx?page=content-subsidi-tf_gender-genderh [accessed 13 December 2011].

Interagency Working Group on Reproductive Health in Crisis (2010) *Interagency Field Manual on Reproductive Health in Humanitarian Settings* [website], 2010 revision for field review http://www.who.int/reproductivehealth/publications/emergencies/field_manual_rh_humanitarian_settings.pdf [accessed 24 August 2011].

IRIN News (2010) *Sanitary Pad Project Changes Lives of DRC Refugees in Uganda* [website], Hopebuilding: Stories at Work http://hopebuilding.pbworks.com/w/page/19222288/Affordable-menstrual-pads-keep-girls-in-school-create-jobs [accessed 30 June 2011].

IRIN News (2011) *Sanitary Pads Keep Girls in School* [website], IRIN http://www.irinnews.org/report.aspx?reportid=93291 [accessed 21 July 2011].

McMahon, S., Winch, J., Caruso, B., Obure, A., Ogutu, E., Ochari, I. and Rheingans, R.D. (2011) 'â€œThe girl with her period is the one to hang her headâ€: Reflections on menstrual management among schoolgirls in rural Kenya', *BMC International Health and Human Rights* 11(7): 1–10.

Mahon, T. and Fernandes, M. (2010) *Menstrual Hygiene in South Asia: A Neglected Issue for WASH Programmes*, WaterAid, London.

Marshall, R. (1995) '(Refugee women) – Refugees, feminine plural', *Refugees Magazine*, Issue 100 [website], UNHCR <http:/www.unhcr.org/3b542be94.html> [accessed 1 August 2011].

MISP (2007) *Minimal Initial Service Package (MISP) for Reproductive Health in Crisis Situations: A Distance Learning Module*, Reproductive Health Rights Consortium, Women's Commission for Refugee Women and Children, New York.

Mutuli, M. and Nyabera, E. (2008) *Chartered Jumbo Jet Flies UNHCR Aid to Kenya* [website], UNHCR http://www.unhcr.org/4790cbc82.html [accessed 1 August 2011].

Nawaz, J., Lal, S., Raza, S. and House, S. (2006) 'Screened toilet, bathing and menstruation units for the earthquake response in NWFP, Pakistan', *WEDC Briefing Paper, 32nd WEDC International Conference*, Sri Lanka.

Nawaz, J., Lal, S. Raza, S. and House, S. (2010) 'Oxfam experience of providing screened toilet, bathing and menstruation units in its earthquake response in Pakistan', *Gender & Development* 18: 81–86.

Oster, E. and Thornton, R. (2009) *Menstruation and Education in Nepal*, Working Paper 14853, National Bureau of Economic Research, Washington, DC.

Proctor & Gamble (2010) *Proctor & Gamble Haiti Earthquake: Touching Lives in Times of Crisis* [website] www.pg.com/sustainability [accessed 27 June 2011].

Scott, L., Dopson, S., Montgomery, P., Dolan, C. and Ryus, C. (2009) *Impact of Providing Sanitary Pads to Poor Girls in Africa*, unpublished report, Oxford University, Oxford.

Shergill, M. (undated) *Hygiene in Emergencies* [website], presentation transcript <http://www.slideshare.net/mshergill/hygieneinemergencies> [accessed 24 August 2011].

Sommer, M. (2009) 'Where the education system and women's bodies collide: The social and health impact of girls' experiences of menstruation and schooling in Tanzania', *Journal of Adolescence* 33(4): 521–529.

Sommer, M. (2010) 'Putting â€œmenstrual hygiene managementâ€ into the school water and sanitation agenda', *Waterlines* 29(4): 268–278, http://dx.doi.org/10.3362/1756-3488.2010.030

Sommer, M. (2011) *Global Review of Menstrual Beliefs and Behaviors in Low-income Countries: Implications for Menstrual Hygiene Management*, unpublished report.

Sphere (2000) *The Sphere Project: Humanitarian charter and minimum standards in humanitarian response* www.sphereproject.org, Oxfam Publishing: Oxford.

Sphere (2004) *The Sphere Project: Humanitarian charter and minimum standards in humanitarian response* www.sphereproject.org, Oxfam Publishig: Oxford.

Sphere (2011) *The Sphere Project: Humanitarian charter and minimum standards in humanitarian response* www.sphereproject.org, Practical Action Publishing, Rugby, UK http://www.developmentbookshelf.com/doi/book/10.3362/9781908176202 [Accessed 22nd May 2015 <http:/dx.doi.org/10.3362/9781908176202>.

UNFPA (2009) *Meeting adolescent sexual and reproductive health needs. Adolescent Sexual and Reproductive Health Toolkit for Humanitarian Settings* http://www.unfpa.org/webdav/site/global/shared/documents/publications/2009/adol_toolkit_humanitarian.pdf [accessed 13 December 2011].

UNHCR (2000) *Country Operation: Yemen*, UNHCR Mid-Year Progress Report 2000 [website] http://www.unhcr.org/3e6f1b870.html [accessed 1 August 2011].

UNHCR (2003) *Country Operations Plan: 2003*, UNHCR, Nairobi, Kenya.

UNHCR (2006) *The UNHCR Tool for Participatory Assessment in Operations*, UNHCR, Geneva.

UNHCR (2008) *Handbook for the Protection of Women and Girls* [website] http://www.unhcr.org/cgi-bin/texis/vtx/search?page=search&docid=47cfa9fe2&query=handbook%20for%20the%20protection [accessed 24 August 2011].

UNHCR (2010) *UNHCR Distributes Vital Aid to Haitian Earthquake Survivors and Hosts* [website] http://www.unhcr.org/4b8411019.html [accessed 1 August 2011].

UNHCR (2011a) *Sanitary Materials: Not Just 'Women's Business'*, UNCHR, Geneva.

UNHCR (2011b) *Protecting Refugee Women: Promoting Gender Equality* [website], Executive Committee of the High Commissioner's Programme, Standing Committee 51st Meeting http://www.unhcr.org/4de4f71a9.pdf [accessed 31 August 2011].

UNHCR (2011c) *WASH not WatSan: Making the Hardware Work Harder*, UNHCR Hygiene Promotion Briefing Pack, unpublished report, UNHCR, Geneva.

UNICEF (2006) *UNICEF Pakistan Earthquake Response*, UNICEF Pakistan Earthquake Response Information Sheet: Water, Environment and Sanitation, UNICEF, Geneva.

WaterAid (2010) 'Menstrual hygiene in South Asia: A neglected issue for WASH programmes', *Gender and Development* 18(1): 99–113.

Women's Commission (2008) *Reproductive Health Coordination Gap, Services Ad Hoc: Minimum Initial Services Package (MISP) Assessment in Kenya*, Women's Commission for Refugee Women and Children, New York.

Websites

IFRC Emergency Items Catalogue 'Hygiene items and parcels' [website], http://procurement.ifrc.org/catalogue/detail.aspx?volume=1&groupcode=108&familycode=108002&categorycode=DIAP&productcode=HHYGPERS02 [accessed 7 August 2011].

IFRC Emergency Items Catalogue 'Hygiene promotion boxes' [website], http://procurement.ifrc.org/catalogue/detail.aspx?volume=1&groupcode=114&familycode=114011&categorycode=HYGP&productcode=KSANHYGP01 [accessed 7 August 2011].

INEE 'Comfort kits', SoE/SBEP Gender Equity Support Program [website], http://toolkit.ineesite.org/toolkit/INEEcms/uploads/1042/Gender_Equity_Strategies_Comfort.PDF [accessed 24 August 2011].

CHAPTER 6

Bulk water treatment unit performance: for the cameras or the community?

Richard Luff and Caetano Dorea

Abstract

As humanitarians we must be deeply concerned about using the most effective solutions for saving lives and reducing morbidity, whilst working within reasonable cost envelopes. In this respect it is critical to place the brightest spotlight upon the practice of using bulk water treatment units (BWTU), as witnessed most recently on a massive scale in the Pakistan floods of 2010. There, as in other huge crises, many BWTUs were deployed by donors and other agencies, sometimes as a knee-jerk reaction to an overwhelming crisis. These appear to offer neat 'plug and play' solutions that also happen to be very media friendly. However, some of the BWTUs sent to flood-affected areas of Pakistan in 2010 demonstrate that there is an absence of appropriate selection criteria for BWTUs and the significant limitations on their use are not fully understood. Though the evidence gathered is partial, there is enough to suggest that some agencies are engaging in poor practice.

Keywords: bulk water treatment units (BWTU); household water treatment and safe storage (HWTS); turbidity; humanitarian water supply

A variety of bulk water treatment units (BWTU), characterized by centralized production of large volumes of water (defined here as 1 to 20 m^3/h), have been used by humanitarian agencies for several decades. There has been field testing and some further development of a few of these in conjunction with manufacturers to provide a package that operates within agency acceptable capital and operating cost envelopes (Dorea et al., 2009; Clarke and Steele, 2010). However there are also many units whose capital and operating costs are far higher, which are too complex to easily operate in crisis conditions, and with unknown field performance. Most manufacturers of BWTUs seek to be able to produce water of the highest possible quality (Luff, 2004) in conformity with European or North American quality standards, focusing their 'sales pitch' mainly on water-borne diseases such as cholera and typhoid. Such technologies typically tend to present a skewed premium on 'instantaneous' or 'plug and play' water systems (i.e. ones requiring minimal operator involvement in installation and operation). Furthermore the centralized production is best suited for large concentrations of static populations, but not all crises fit this scenario.

http://dx.doi.org/10.3362/9781780448831.006

On close analysis this treatment option does not fit with requirements for water supply in many humanitarian situations and alternatives are available. For example, simple batch chlorination can be an appropriate, reliable, and well-practised treatment where water is not turbid (i.e. ideally less than 5 nephelometric turbidity units, NTU) and the presence of chlorination-resistant protozoan pathogens is unlikely (e.g. groundwater). However, surface water sources are often the most accessible source available and often contain high (i.e. more than 50 NTU) levels of turbidity, which can be one of the greatest challenges in emergency water treatment. As a result, the use of BWTUs is warranted. However, many of the commercially available BWTUs seem to be primarily equipped to deal with microbiological and sometimes chemical contamination, but not to deal with high levels of turbidity. This is a significant fact, since the water treatment yield of such units typically drops off significantly when dealing with turbidities over 50 to 100 NTU (ICRC, 1995; Dorea et al., 2009). Yet, emergency response guidelines suggest that the supply of large quantities of relatively clean water have greater positive impact on diarrhoeal disease reduction than limited quantities of very pure (and frequently more expensive) water (Smith and Reed, 1991; The Sphere Project, 2011). This indicates that there may be deficiencies in the design and also in the selection of certain BWTUs. Whilst the design of such units concerns manufacturers, their selection by agencies merits appraisal and is the objective of this article.

BWTU selection and deployment criteria

In order to make sense of whether and when BWTUs should be purchased and used in an emergency, it is necessary to be clear about what is really required and what has proved effective in addressing the affected population's public health needs. To this end, four criteria that should be considered during the selection (or not) of BWTUs for deployment have been identified:

- event duration and population densities;
- capital costs and simplicity;
- focus on turbidity not purity;
- independent testing and verification.

Event duration and population densities

Some crises, such as armed conflict and urban earthquakes, tend to create concentrations of people in camp-like situations for longer periods of time. In these situations, where there is a high static population density, there may be a role for BWTUs, as the requirement will typically be for centralized water treatment and distribution systems to be set up. However, other catastrophic events such as floods and cyclones can often create short-term displacements where people are able to return to their homes within days or weeks.

Table 6.1 Water treatment options based on anticipated displacement duration and affected population characteristics*

Anticipated duration of displacement crisis	Population size and concentration	Proposed drinking water treatment options
1–6 weeks, e.g. rural floods/cyclones	Dispersed in their villages	Household water treatment
1–6 weeks, e.g. rural floods/cyclones	Displaced on high areas of ground e.g. embankments in groups of up to 3,000–6,000	1) Household water treatment 2) Very simple BWTU 1,000–2,000 l/h
8–12 weeks, e.g. floods	Schools and IDP camps for 5,000 people plus	1) BWTU 2,000–10,000 l/h 2) Simple batch water treatment in camps
3–15 months, e.g. for longer-term conflict and earthquake displaced	Large tented camps for 5,000 people plus	1) BWTU 2,000–10,000 l/h 2) Simple batch water treatment in camps

Note: *Assumptions:

- The source will be flood water and around 3 to 4 litres of drinking water per person per day of treated water needs to be supplied.
- Water for anal cleansing and bathing will not necessarily be treated.
- Provision of separate supplies of potable water and water for other purposes can be managed through additional household water containers, additional bulk water tanks, and hygiene promotion. Though this is more complex to arrange, treating all water using BWTUs is considered much more complicated and costly.

When dealing with dispersed and mobile populations, these situations in particular pose significant challenges in reaching the victims and the reality is that often they have to fend for themselves, as water from BWTUs simply can't reach them. Decentralized interventions, such as household water treatment and storage (HWTS), can have a far greater 'reach' by providing means by which people can treat water themselves. Therefore, different situations will demand different interventions. To this end, experienced staff using initial assessments should make judgements with regard to the necessary interventions. Given the varied nature of disasters, one type of response may not always conform to each situation. However, albeit non-exhaustive in terms of scenarios, guidance examples with regard to water treatment options are provided in Table 6.1.

Capital costs and simplicity

The range of capital costs for emergency BWTUs is extremely broad (Luff, 2004; Simpson and Dorea, 2010). If we argue that emphasis should be placed on the provision of large volumes of adequate quality water, as opposed to small quantities of highly pure water, it follows that BWTU capital costs can be further evaluated in terms of their cost per production capacity yield (US$/m3/h). A full cost-benefit analysis is beyond the scope of this article and different agencies have varied views about what an upper cost threshold should be for BWTUs. Nonetheless, some BWTUs can be considered extremely expensive costing up to $12,000/m3/h (of claimed production capacity). This is in stark contrast with other units costing $2,000/m^3/h, which may still be considered high, but is in the lower range of costs and is definitely more affordable. Experience has shown that capital costs are typically a proxy for the complexity of the BWTU. High-cost units are in general more sophisticated with a focus on extreme water purity and not quantity. Furthermore, having more low-cost units in place of fewer expensive ones, could build in further flexibility and robustness to a water supply strategy. It is suggested that high cost and complexity preclude some units from ever being suitable for deployment and a closer examination of this is required to determine an upper cost threshold.

Turbidity not purity

One aspect of water treatment overlooked by many BWTU manufacturers is how such units deal with very high levels of turbidly (Luff, 2004). The focus of many units is to deal with microbiological purity and chemical contamination, presumably in order to meet developed world water quality standards, as this may also be a market for many manufacturers. The choice of treatment process typically reflects this focus at the cost of production yield and often results in technologies that do not cope well with field conditions they might be expected to encounter during emergencies, such as high turbidities experienced during floods. That is, many BWTUs are not addressing the quantity vs. quality criteria discussed earlier and often utilize sophisticated filtration-based processes that, when faced with turbidity challenges, will quickly clog up, resulting in a rapid drop off in production capacity. This was evident in the interagency trials of a range of equipment in Geneva in 1995 (ICRC, 1995) and field observations. Nonetheless, many manufacturers of BWTUs:

- have failed to have made adequate provision for coping with suspended solids in the design;
- have focused on high levels of water purity to standards that are not demanded in many countries affected by crises (The Sphere Project, 2011);
- provide no testing and data on how such units perform over a range of turbidities.

The fact that so many BWTUs are purchased/supplied by donors/agencies without taking into account these very clear concerns is highly problematic.

Independent testing and verification

It remains a major concern that a variety of organizations continue to purchase BWTUs without clear criteria based upon field realities supported by independent testing and verification. At this stage a thorough, up-to-date survey of which manufacturers provide independent testing and verification has not been undertaken. Frequently, the extent of reported testing is very limited and where undertaken it is linked primarily to microbiological water purity. Independent verification of claimed rates of production, how these continue over periods of weeks and months, performance for a range of turbidities, operational cost, and complexities are the critical aspects that need examining. Work on cost effectiveness, which looks at actual production rates over several weeks versus capital and operational costs, also needs to be considered. This sort of data is critical for agencies to make objective decisions about BWTU purchase.

A challenge for suppliers of BWTUs is to know what criteria to design and test their units against as a set of sector-wide agreed criteria does not exist. While levels of expenditure on these units were significant in Pakistan and elsewhere, there are no moves under way at this time for agencies to agree sector-wide criteria. However, this is the single most important step the major agencies must take in order to reduce wasteful and inappropriate expenditure. Donors should also make it a requirement that any purchased BWTUs conform to such criteria.

A comparison between BWTUs and HWTS

Table 6.1 exemplified flooding situations where the use of emergency HWTS could be considered as an alternative to the use of BWTUs. There are major challenges with use of HWTS (Clasen et al., 2006) and this is not to suggest that this is panacea to water quality challenges in crisis situations. Nonetheless it may be instructive to compare both of these by considering costs and some of the assumptions about the way in which they are utilized.

The costs for use of BWTUs are very uncertain for a number of reasons. Some assumptions are made for the purpose of the estimate.

- Duration of need and thus potential use for BWTUs is very uncertain. It is suggested above that use should be targeted at those who are displaced as they tend to be the most vulnerable, while populations returning to their homes should have assistance though provision of long-term solutions. For many flood situations, up to 1 month of displacement would be likely, though floods in Pakistan were exceptional and many people remained displaced for 2–3 months.
- As explained above, BWTUs have inherent limitations which make them an inflexible option and it is often the case that the full production capacity is not utilized. However for the purpose of this exercise it is assumed that demand equals or exceeds capacity so all water produced can be targeted at those in need.
- If the units have single use, then all capital costs have to be allocated to the population served. Some agencies may take such units back to their

Table 6.2 Characteristics of an LMS unit deployed to Pakistan in 2010

Capital cost for LMS unit	$45,000
Stated production rate of	15 m³/h
Assumed operation time, which allows down time for cleaning/maintenance	8 hours
Over a 30 day period this would produce	3.6 million litres
120 litres potable water/person/month used from the units (4 l/person/day)	$1.5/person/month

home country, while others may donate them to local governments. In the latter case, whether these get used again is a major question because they are at times so specialized often requiring external parts and expertise in order to use them.

Table 6.2 shows an example of one unit (the 'LMS' unit) used quite extensively over the years in different crises, using the assumptions set out above.

This cost does not factor in maintenance and consumables, or flights/transportation/accommodation costs for international staff, which could easily add another 15–30 per cent on top of these costs.

To the authors' knowledge, though this is not a direct comparison that has been made before, examining HWTS as an alternative in areas where populations are dispersed and in smaller camps for shorter durations is significant because it starts to look at efficiency from a cost perspective. HWTS distributions to populations are certainly higher risk as it is known that bulk distribution of packages of HWTS options without hygiene promotion will result in low levels of correct utilization. However, while not common practice, studies have shown there are a couple of critical factors that maximize efficacy:

- Prior knowledge of product is very helpful and makes the task of hygiene promotion easier.
- For options that the population are not familiar with, refresher training to follow up initial training is an important factor to significantly improve correct uptake.

Data from a recent study on use of HWTS in emergencies conducted by Daniele Lantagne (LSHTM) on behalf of UNICEF and Oxfam is summarized in Table 6.3.

It has to be noted that the LMS does have the capacity to deal with high turbidity (i.e. > 50 NTU), while clearly people would have to deal with any turbidity in their water prior to the use of chlorine products, perhaps through low-cost options such as sedimentation and/or straining water through a cloth (Kotlarz et al., 2009; Preston et al., 2010). (Ceramic filters or combined coagulant disinfectant can be used to deal with higher turbidity water.)

While BWTUs need high levels of technical support and certain conditions for optimum use, Table 6.3 shows that HWTS options require good

Table 6.3 Summary of costs of different HWTS

	Single training	Follow-up training	Cost/year/ person	Cost/month/ person
PuR	10–54%	89–95.4%	US$0.39	US$0.03
Hypochlorite	3–25%	76%	US$0.06	US$0.005
Ceramics	26.3%		US$0.25	US$0.02

Source: Lantagne and Clasen (2009)

Note: Costs based on a bottle of hypochlorite treating 1,000 litres (average $0.33), a sachet of PuR 10 litres ($0.35), and a tablet 20 litres ($0.01). We use a family using 20 litres per day (5 people, 4 litres each) in this table. % effective use as measured at household level.

hygiene promotion and use messaging with follow up in order to be used effectively by households, especially where the treatment technology is unfamiliar. The programme costs of this would also need to be computed for a more representative comparison between the different modes of water treatment. However a straight capital cost comparison shows that certain BWTUs can be much more expensive per litre than some HWTS options. If the LMS unit was used for over 8 years, its costs are comparable to use of ceramic filters. In the absence of a more informed study, this comparison can only reveal the order of magnitude difference in costs and as such should demand much greater scrutiny before BWTUs are purchased in future. It also highlights the importance of a more informed study to look at costs more closely.

However, it is important to look not just at costs but also the risk of the benefits of investments not being realized. BWTUs can be high-risk investments because their deployment comes with a number of hidden assumptions which are often not taken into account:

- They have to be near to populations they serve, i.e. they don't have much 'reach'.
- Their levels of utilization are uncertain and for the larger units it is rare for demand to match *required* potable water supply (3 l/person/day).
- Their use post-crisis is seldom followed up and their viability for subsequent use without high levels of external support is in doubt; although this is not always the case (Dorea et al., 2009).

HWTS options can be much more versatile where they are deployed and thus have greater reach and lower risk. They also offer protection of water quality at point of consumption, thereby reducing risk of recontamination after treatment. These options need to be supported with initial and follow-up training programmes in order to have higher levels of efficacy than many have had to date. There is certainly much more work to be undertaken to deliver more certain results for HWTS programmes in emergencies but the options available are both more flexible and in line with longer-term development thinking.

BWTUs in the 2010 Pakistan floods

The floods in Pakistan affected large parts of the country, initially in the north in early August 2010, then flooding massive areas of land primarily in the Punjab and Sindh provinces over the following couple of months. Huge numbers of people were affected and significant numbers were displaced and occupied areas of high land, road embankments and schools and later were put in tent camps of a few hundred to several thousands of people. OCHA situation reports (14 August 2010 to 14 September 2010) exemplify and highlight the rise in total numbers of flood-affected victims (14.5 to 20 million) and numbers of displaced people in Sindh province (0.3 to 1.4 million) in the span of a month. These numbers also reflect the victims who might be presumed to be located where BWTUs could have a role to play.

Already by mid-to-late August there was a growing sense that the scale of this crisis was completely overwhelming for a number of reasons: the sheer numbers of people reported as affected; the extent of flooding right across the country; and hydrological predictions that flood water would remain for a few months particularly in Sindh province. It is worth noting that sometimes greater numbers of people have been reported as affected by floods in parts of China and India in the previous decade, but these have not invoked the same sense of overwhelming need and international response.

This scale of crisis, which demanded a massive response, attracted significant levels of international attention, and understandably invoked calls for assistance from all quarters. On 25 August, UNICEF, with support from WHO (WASH and health cluster leads, respectively), called for an urgent extraordinary joint appeal for WASH items, amongst which was the request for 30 water purification units with capacity between 5,000 and 15,000 litres per hour. Suppliers, when approached with a request based upon these vague criteria, were understandably only too willing to provide their equipment where funds were forthcoming. This request was in addition to some BWTUs that had already been deployed to Pakistan by a variety of government donors and UN/NGOs. Given this was such an urgent, high-level request and there are no sector-wide criteria to determine which BWTUs are suitable, it was unsurprising that many totally unsuitable units were supplied, alongside other units that can perform well in the right conditions.

Table 6.4 gives an overview of BWTUs deployed in Pakistan. It is compiled from the knowledge of one of the authors from his deployment to Pakistan in late August 2010, from WASH cluster information, and e-mail correspondence with donors, suppliers and NGOs, among others. Some BWTU costs and numbers have been verified with manufacturers, but many manufacturers either did not respond when asked to corroborate or we did not have their contact details. Where information is marked as NA (not available) it has either proved impossible to track down or some suppliers have been unwilling to provide it. It should be noted that in addition to BWTUs, HWTS options, chlorination, drilling boreholes and so on were all provided, but in the authors' experience of working in major crises for over 20 years, the scale of deployment of BWTUs to Pakistan is unequalled.

Table 6.4 Overview of BWTUs reported to WASH cluster as deployed in response to Pakistan floods in first three months (Aug–Oct 2010)

Purchasing organization	Implementing/ operation agency	Unit type/ model	No. deployed	Purchase cost ($) i.e. per unit	Manufacturers rated capacity (m³/h)
Gov Luxembourg	UNICEF	RO unit with max capacity	1	$569,897	NA
Swedish Gov?	UNICEF	NA	1	$892,806	NA
NA	UNICEF	NA	1	$21,418	NA
NA	UNICEF	NA	2	$93,677	NA
DFID	HANDICAP, Muslim Aid, IRC, IRD	Large purification unit	5	NA	NA
DFID	NRSP, IRC	Small purification unit	2	NA	NA
DFID	UNICEF – then to WASH cluster	Aquacube VT-100	2	£55,000	288m³/day
DFID	UNICEF – then to WASH cluster	Aquacube MT	1	£15,000	10
USAID	UNICEF	Trailer mounted LMS units (OX-A3)	7	$44,353	15
USAID	Gov. Pakistan	Trailer mounted LMS units (OX-A3)	6	$44,353	15
German Gov	PHED	NA	NA	NA	2–6
UNICEF	Aqua assistance/ UNICEF	Aquatech	3	$60,000	5
UNICEF	NA	Aqua units	NA	$16,000	4
UNICEF	PHED	Sosafe	6	NA	5–6
UNICEF	PHED	Tauseefwater	19	NA	2
MSB	MSB	NA	10	NA	1.2
Gov of France	PHED	NA	3		10
Gov China	NDMA (Pakistan National Disaster Management Authority)	Some RO units	49	NA	NA
IFRC	Pakistan Red Crescent Society	2 units	NA	NA	NA

(Continued)

Table 6.4 Overview of BWTUs reported to WASH cluster as deployed in response to Pakistan floods in first three months (Aug–Oct 2010) (Continued)

Purchasing organization	Implementing/ operation agency	Unit type/ model	No. deployed	Purchase cost ($) i.e. per unit	Manufacturers rated capacity (m³/h)
Spanish Red Cross	Spanish Red Cross	NA	2	$15,000	NA
German THW	THW	Possibly Berkefeld units	2	NA	6
Various NGOs and Red Cross	Various NGOs and Red Cross	Scanwater EmWat 4000	20	EUR 14,915	4
NA	NA	Scanwater TEW 202D	1	EUR 29,590	20
NCA	CERD/Sungi	NA	2	NA	NA
Total			145	$3.14 m	

There are a variety of units specified here and though this paper does not seek to comment on relative performance and appropriateness of the various units, some are quite simply totally unsuitable for such conditions and should never have been sent. However it is important to again highlight that some donors and agencies have many years' experience of BWTUs and make purchase choices based upon their own criteria. For example the LMS units have been used over a period of more than 15 years and have evolved through a process of agency feedback based upon programme experience.

The operational complexities and limitations (Dorea et al., 2009) of these units are not captured in this table, but there are a number of critical aspects that need to be highlighted:

- Treatment/pumping/backwashing complexity requires many of these units to be operated by specialist teams, either on a short-term basis and handed over to national operatives or for the more complex (expensive units) by dedicated teams of international staff. The costs of dedicated international staff (flights/transport/per diems etc.) are usually significant.
- Deployment of international staff in insecure locations (i.e. much of Pakistan) is highly problematic. In late August 2010 so-called Taliban groups announced they would target relief workers specifically.
- Unless BWTUs are set up in or adjacent to a camp/IDP centre where water can be piped to populations, they are dependent upon water trucks to move water, so their 'reach' can be limited.

The suitability of some of these units in any situation is questionable and the deployment of so many (145 units at average production of 5,000 litres/h could optimistically serve 1.9 million people at 3 litres of water per person/

day) is highly questionable. As explained above, the 'reach' and complexity can make their use extremely limited and the costs for some units sent should be viewed as prohibitive in all but specialized situations such as water supply to hospitals where the highest purity of water is required.

At the stage of data collection in late August there was very little data coming to the central WASH cluster information systems, but some feedback provided by five different agencies who were directly involved in using BWTUs is set out below:

- With reference to the unit provided by the Luxembourg Government, the feedback highlights the significant additional costs associated with supporting the deployment of the BWTU over and above the capital cost. It also points out that high turbidity and security limited operating time and thus considerably reduced claimed/optimum output: '€2–3 m + $35,000 given to UNICEF to cover accommodation and living costs of the nine military staff installing this BWTU which comes with a Mercedes jeep + two trucks. It operates at 17,000 litres/hour due to high turbidity, security restrictions and the 4 hrs down time for filter cleaning per day.'
- This comment was shared in response to BWTUs in general and highlights that BWTUs are/or become redundant when there are alternative water sources: 'Some are – just for filling tankers but even then most of our tankers now fill up from deep boreholes. When it is, for the majority of places, so easy, quick and cheap to install a borehole with hand pump – which is what the people want, then Pakistan is just another of the numerous examples of why water treatment units are not only rarely effective but waste so much money'.
- In the case of RO units provided by the Chinese Government, the absence of a generator in the kits meant users, in this case Pakistan water authorities, needed to also find generators to power these units where remoteness of location/damage to power lines meant main power was not available, again limiting their flexibility: 'These units required electric power supply, no generators are included in kits'.
- This comment highlighted that some capacity was either redundant from the start or not deployed to the right location, while the availability of water truck capacity is a prerequisite in all situations except that outlined above: '1 Unit not used at all while the other unit had no distribution capacity to truck water out from water production points to the affected population'.
- Again the problems of high turbidity are so often not acknowledged, let alone addressed by manufacturers, which in this case meant the unit was only able to produce a mere 15 per cent of stated capacity. In essence this meant water would cost 6.6 times the amount that might have been presumed from manufacturers rating without pre-treatment: 'In general very positive. National engineers were able to install and operate. Main problem is raw water very silt laden. Plant throughput re-rated to

15 per cent of name plate capacity. However high quality finished water achievable at greatly reduced rate. Now installing 5,000 litre sedimentation tanks upstream to knock out the heaviest silt – should allow greater throughput but consider name plate rating optimistic and only achievable under ideal conditions.'

Data from a HWTS study following the 2009 earthquake in Indonesia (Lantagne and Clasen, 2011) broadened the study focus to include researching small-scale water treatment units and found that 38 water treatment units were registered by 17 NGOs in the first 3 weeks after crisis onset. One agency staff person responded: 'how we ensure that people are not flying in with the things that are not appropriate' as 'having thousands of, millions of Aquatabs coming in which is not necessary' and 'having people coming with purification units and they only have three days to install it and go' are of no utility, especially because 'too much equipment that will be left behind and not used because they don't know how to use or they don't have the chemicals for it.'

Conclusions

The critical points that can be drawn out from the Pakistan and global (e.g. Haiti, Indonesia, Bangladesh, and others) experience are:

- An excessive number of BWTUs were deployed to Pakistan, owing to hasty decision-making in response to a massive crisis and in response to the WASH cluster request.
- Some BWTUs deployed were a waste of money as they were too expensive and complex, certainly for this and probably for most contexts.
- BWTUs are the wrong solution for short-term displacements of large numbers of people over large areas as was the case for the majority of people in Pakistan.
- BWTUs have significant direct operational costs and indirect costs associated with tying up staff, for which there is little information available and which is not accounted for. HWTS is less high tech and can be supported without specialized staff and equipment.
- There is an absence of sector-wide agreed selection criteria that can be used by purchasers of BWTUs to ensure that inappropriate and wasteful choices are not repeated.
- While suppliers/manufacturers of BWTUs will naturally respond to purchase orders for their units, they must be made more accountable by being required to undertake independent testing and verification of their units under realistically simulated programme conditions and make future purchase by relief agencies conditional upon this.
- Household water treatment and safe storage options (HWTS) are cheaper and likely to be more cost effective as they can have much greater flexibility in highly unpredictable crisis situations.

Recommendations

Given the significant levels of expenditure on BWTUs, there should be a sector-wide review undertaken by the major organizations that purchase and use BWTUs – donors, NGOs, and the UN to:

- Develop criteria for unit selection and agree these sector-wide (this should also include any offers for goods in kind – GiK). This article proposes criteria as the basis for this work.
- Make any future purchase of BWTUs conditional upon manufacturers having undertaken (and paid for) independent testing and verification of their units.
- Undertake a more thorough study of costs and effectiveness between BWTUs and HWTS options.

About the authors

Richard Luff (richardluff06@googlemail.com) is a chartered health engineer with over 20 years' experience working for UNICEF, Oxfam and DFID as a humanitarian specialist. **Caetano Dorea** is a professor in the Département de génie civil et de génie des eaux, Université Laval, Quebec, Canada.

References

Clarke, B.A. and Steele, A. (2010) 'Water treatment systems for relief agencies: The on-going search for the "Silver Bullet"', *Desalination* 251: 64–71.

Clasen, T., Smith, L., Albert, J., Bastable, A. and Fesselet, J. (2006) 'The drinking water response to the Indian Ocean tsunami, including the role of household water treatment', *Disaster Prevention & Management* 15(1): 190–201, http://dx.doi.org/10.1108/09653560610654338

Dorea, C.C., Luff, R., Bastable, A. and Clarke, B.A. (2009) 'Up-flow clarifier for emergency water treatment', *Water and Environment Journal* 23(4): 293–299, http://dx.doi.org/10.1111/j.1747-6593.2008.00142.x

ICRC (1995) *Interagency Technical Meeting: Water Treatment Units*, unpublished report, ICRC, Geneva.

Kotlarz N., Lantagne D., Preston K. and Jellison K. (2009) 'Turbidity and chlorine demand reduction using locally available physical water clarification mechanisms before household chlorination in developing countries' *Journal of Water and Health*, 7(3):497–506.

Lantagne, D. and Clasen, T. (2009) *Point-of-Use Water Treatment in Emergency Response*, London School of Hygiene and Tropical Medicine, London.

Lantagne, D. and Clasen, T. (2011) *Assessing the Implementation of Selected Household Water Treatment and Safe Storage Methods in Emergency Settings*, London School of Hygiene and Tropical Medicine, London.

Luff, R. (2004) 'Paying too much for Purity', paper presented to WEDC annual conference, Vientiane, Oct 2004.

Preston, K., Lantagne, D., Kotlarz, N. and Jellison, K. (2010) 'Turbidity and chlorine demand reduction using alum and moringa flocculation before household chlorination in developing countries', *Journal of Water and Health* 8(1): 60–70, http://dx.doi.org/10.2166/wh.2009.210

Simpson, M.R. and Dorea, C.C. (2010) 'Cost-effectiveness of emergency water treatment kits', in *1st International Conference of Disaster Prevention Technology and Management (DPTM-2010)*, 23–25 October 2010, Chonqing, China.

Smith, M. and Reed, R. (1991) 'Water and sanitation for disasters', *Tropical Doctor* 21: 30–37.

The Sphere Project (2011) *Humanitarian Charter and Minimum Standards in Disaster Response*, Practical Action Publishing, Rugby, UK http://www.developmentbookshelf.com/doi/book/10.3362/9781908176202 [Accessed 22nd May 2015 <http:/dx.doi.org/10.3362/9781908176202>.

CHAPTER 7

Innovative designs and approaches in sanitation when responding to challenging and complex humanitarian contexts in urban areas

Andy Bastable and Jenny Lamb

Abstract

As recent emergencies have shown, there are still significant challenges in the timely provision of safe sanitation in natural disasters or conflict situations. In urban emergencies or areas where it is impossible to dig simple pit latrines because of high water tables, hard rock, or lack of permission, it takes agencies considerable time to construct elevated latrines or alternative designs such as urine diversion toilets. This paper describes the challenges often faced in the rapid construction of latrines in emergencies and then looks at a number of case studies, from the Haiti earthquake and the 2010 floods in the Philippines, of how these obstacles were overcome. It also documents some of the recent innovations and improvements suppliers have made in increasing the scope of their emergency sanitation equipment.

Keywords: pit latrines, urine-diverting latrines, humanitarian sanitation

Over the last couple of years, there has been an array of natural disasters, which have led to massive levels of destruction, loss of life, and disorder. Humanitarian agencies are increasingly responding to more frequent disasters in urban areas, such as in Haiti, the Philippines, and Pakistan (although the latter less so for urban areas). The earthquake that struck Haiti had a devastating impact, leaving more than a million homeless, killing more than 220,000 people and injuring over 300,000 people. The death toll in Pakistan was lower: more than 1,750 people are thought to have died; however the number of people affected by the flood was huge, in the region of 21 million people.

On the first day of the response, a humanitarian worker will review their contingency stocks, open their logistics equipment catalogue and order a cargo plane jam-packed full of water and sanitation materials. When you make your shopping list of equipment for water supply, there is an array of materials to chose from, whereas for sanitation there will simply be the squatting latrine slab, plastic sheeting, and hygiene promotion materials and equipment.

http://dx.doi.org/10.3362/9781780448831.007

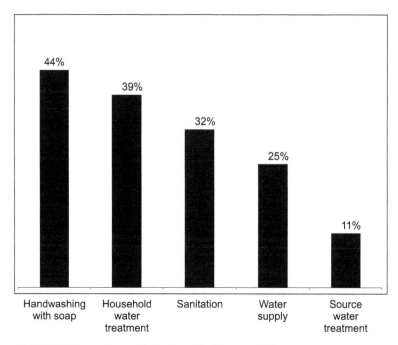

Figure 7.1 WASH interventions which reduce diarrhoea morbidity
Source: adapted from Fewtrell et al. (2005)

Fewtrell et al. (2005) provide informative conclusions on which WASH intervention significantly reduces diarrhoea morbidity. In order of significance, hand washing, has the highest impact at 44 per cent, sanitation 32 per cent, and water supply 25 per cent (Figure 7.1).

Given the conclusions from Fewtrell et al., the lack of diversity of equipment to respond to sanitation in emergencies, and the increased challenges faced when implementing sanitation in urban areas, there is the need, now more than ever, to increase the range of appropriate sanitation equipment. However, this should not be done in isolation of hand washing, the intervention which has the greatest impact on reducing diarrhoea morbidity. Currently, it appears that there is an inverse relationship between money spent and effectiveness at reducing diarrhoea: currently the majority of spend is on water supply and quality, rather than hand washing, public health promotion, and safe sanitation.

So, what can we do to increase our effectiveness in responding to sanitation in emergencies, and how can we bring hand washing up to an equal footing with water and sanitation?

The case studies in the next section highlight the challenges in responding in urban areas, and will furthermore offer recommendations for agencies, donors, local authorities, and communities on what they should be engaged with and prioritizing. It should also be noted that some of these recommendations are already being implemented through outputs from the Sanitation Interagency Meeting at Stoutenburg, Netherlands. For instance, agencies including Oxfam

GB are working in conjunction with key suppliers to experiment and build sanitation prototypes to fill this gap and respond effectively to the need for sanitation equipment appropriate for emergencies.

Context analysis: Challenges in urban areas, case studies from Haiti, Pakistan, and the Philippines

For many years the major challenge for emergency sanitation was the rapid installation of raised latrines in flooded or high water table areas and hard rock sites. It takes time to source and build the raised platform, which makes each latrine twice the price of a normal pit latrine. Another common issue which delays the speedy provision of latrines is unstable soils where again it is time consuming and expensive to provide quick linings to prevent pit or trench collapse. In the last 2 years there has been an increase in these excreta disposal challenges in a response to emergencies in urban areas. The most notable examples are the floods in Greater Manila, the Philippines, in 2009, the Haiti earthquake in Port au Prince in 2010 and some of the areas affected by the Pakistan floods in 2010. The challenge in these urban areas is not only the extra time required to build raised latrines in areas where pit latrines are not feasible but also that in a dense, crowded city ensuring regular desludging can be a major challenge. Lastly, very few cities in developing countries have properly functioning waste treatment plants so by increasing the burden on the various 'sewage ponds' there is a major risk of causing environmental pollution. While the challenges described above mainly concern the rapid installation of emergency latrines, use and maintenance are also considerable challenges in any emergency. Urban displaced populations tend to be less homogeneous, making it more difficult to set up community management committees as one would in a rural setting. While NGOs tend towards paying latrine attendants in these situations this can become difficult to sustain in the long term. Also, while people tend to expect that after the first phase of the emergency they can return to their previous practice of buying water, this is not the case for excreta disposal. Agencies in Haiti today still have huge desludging bills to support the displaced people in camps, who are clearly unable to meet these costs and cater for all their own sanitation needs.

Haiti earthquake

In Haiti, pre-earthquake, only 29 per cent of urban dwellers used improved sanitation (JMP, 2008), with open defecation and flying toilets common in high-density urban areas. The options Oxfam GB considered in Port au Prince, Haiti, were based on the ability to dig into the soil, access for desludging, existing practices, and speed of installation. The first phase options were simple pit latrines where we were able to dig into the soil, 'Portaloos' from areas we were not able to dig, and biodegradable bags. Options which came on line a little later were the raised latrines and large volume septic tanks where we were able to dig. The information below gives some feedback on the various options.

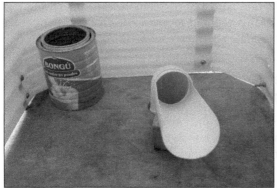 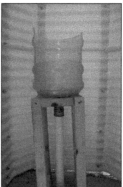

Figure 7.2 Examples of female and male urinals
© Jane Beesley, OGB

Chemical toilets (Portaloos). Chemical toilets hired from private companies were used in some camps. However, given the limited size of the storage capacity and high maintenance cost (over US$20/day initially that went down to $9/day) for emptying/cleaning, their use was quickly discontinued. Some six months after the earthquake, Action Contre la Faim had a monthly desludging bill for the chemical toilets of $500,000. The users expressed their aversion to using these toilets because they could see each other's excreta, and the prevailing heat made them hot inside. Later on, unused Portaloo units were used as showers in Corail: toilet tanks were removed, and the superstructures were installed on concrete foundations to become shower cubicles.

Raised latrine units. Fitted above plastic water tanks, these were used at sites where space was limited, where it was impossible to dig, or where landowners refused permission to dig. The raised latrines required regular desludging by vacuum tankers. Oxfam GB had lower O&M costs than other organizations that opted for Portaloos, as the raised latrine water tank units required desludging every fortnight or once per month. The best configuration was to have 3–4 cubicles discharging into one larger 'water' tank.

Biodegradable bags. Bags, including PeePoo, biodegradable, and simple plastic bags were piloted at two camps where it was impossible to install latrines quickly. Although there were limitations, it did build on people's existing practices (use of plastic bags as 'flying toilets'). The elderly, less physically able and women particularly appreciated PeePoo bags, as these could be used at night in their tents. Use of an organized bag collection system also prevented bags being discarded indiscriminately into drainage channels and ravines.

In particular, PeePoo bags were liked for their ability to reduce smells, especially when used inside tents. Unfortunately, after the initial pilot, bag use was discontinued and an opportunity to provide vulnerable individuals with a 'safe' night toilet option was lost.

Consideration of the users wishing to only urinate, and not defecate, led to some creative thinking: would they want to use a bag or urinate elsewhere? Urinals were designed and implemented for both the men and the women.

INNOVATIVE DESIGNS AND APPROACHES IN SANITATION 101

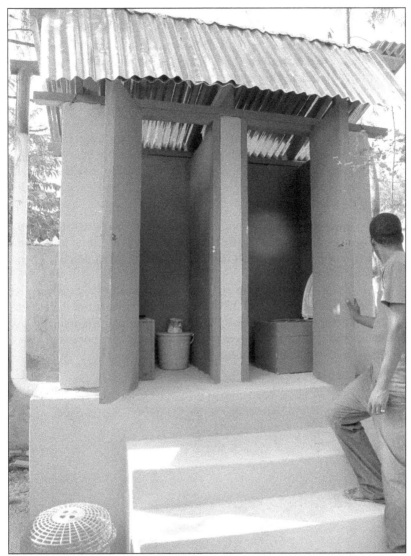

Figure 7.3 Raised urine-diverting toilet units installed and operated by Oxfam's partner, SOIL

Urine diversion (UD) toilets. Oxfam's partner, SOIL, piloted UD toilets at 32 sites, with 194 units installed. The UD toilets differ from routine eco-san latrines in that the urine was diverted to a soak pit, the faeces collected in a drum, and bagasse, a waste product from a local sugar factory, is added after each use (as a drying agent). Two community composting sites were also set up. The pilot worked well owing to the partner's high motivation and community mobilization work. Twelve months on, many of the units are still in operation. Paid toilet attendants, on daily labour rates, is one factor ensuring high user satisfaction with the units.

Regarding anal cleansing, our expectations were that Haitians used tissue paper, but where this was unavailable, or affordable, some people used stones or corn husks for anal cleansing. This caused problems with desludging, as stones and the husks damaged the inlet of the desludging hose, and resulted in the pits filling up quicker than anticipated.

Petion Ville Golf Course: A phased approach

The golf course was the largest camp in Port-au-Prince with a population of 50,000 at the height of the crisis. Given the difficulty of the terrain (limited access for trucks, steep slopes, and rocky ground), a phased approach to excreta disposal was implemented over a year-long period. Latrines were manually desludged on a periodic basis.

- *Phase I*. Emergency latrines built over trenches, using self-supporting slabs, wooden frames and plastic sheeting. In total, 472 drop holes were installed (approx 1:100), with dedicated cubicles for children and the less physically able.
- *Phase II*. Latrines built over deep trenches stabilized by GI (galvanized iron) sheets. Self-supporting slabs and rigid superstructures were used. 472 drop holes were maintained (including cubicles for children and less physically able). Camp members painted the latrines to stimulate better hygiene practices amongst users.

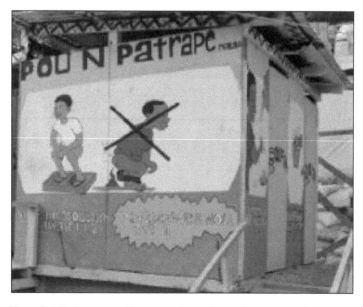

Figure 7.4 Hygiene promotion messaging on the walls to promote better hygiene practices © Kateryna Perus, OGB

- *Phase III*. Latrines were upgraded by building over high volume 50 m³ pits (blocks, reinforcing bar, and concrete). Sit-down seats replaced squatting slabs, and superstructures were made from plywood; 307 drop holes were fitted to high volume pits (including cubicles for children and the less physically able), and again painted by camp members.

2010 Pakistan floods

Shallow trench latrines. Construction of household latrines was impossible for many families because of the technically difficult conditions (high ground water table and availability of material). People were defecating in a fenced area in the compound and then flushing the excreta into a drain or else throwing it outside their compound with the aid of a shovel. To meet the need for an appropriate sanitation option Oxfam GB introduced the idea of shallow trench latrines. The shallow trench latrines were very well received, with comments from women such as: 'This is very good idea. We never thought of it. Now we don't need to go outside or need to wait for dark to relieve ourselves'.

Public health promoters continued working with women and girls on use and maintenance of trench latrines. The demonstration and construction of trench latrines continued in 13 Union Councils of two districts, whereby the team managed to construct more than 6,000 latrines in just 2 months.

Open defecation clean-up campaigns. When Oxfam GB first arrived, some of the camps proved to be very challenging environments: open defecation was rife and in each camp there was a diverse range of ethnic and clan origins. Oxfam GB placed enormous emphasis on community mobilization, and dedicated a great deal of time to discussing the importance of appropriate safe excreta disposal with the camp population. The Oxfam GB team, with their local partners, carried out regular open defecation clean-up campaigns. This required a great deal of dedicated community mobilization, as some were reluctant to clean up the opposing clan's faecal matter. Thereafter, the latrine strategy included shallow trench latrines, pit latrines, and septic tanks, and in some instances pre-identified areas for safe open defecation which the men preferred to use.

Floods in the Philippines

In the Philippines, Oxfam GB used a number of 1 m³ tanks behind raised platforms in densely packed urban situations where digging in was impossible. One of the innovations here was an overflow tank from which the effluent would be desludged, and effectively the system acted like a mini septic tank.

Hand washing with soap. As previously mentioned there is a 44 per cent reduction in morbidity by diarrhoeal disease due to hand washing with soap. As part of our response to Haiti, Pakistan, and the Philippines, hand washing devices were equipped in each camp setting, either through small 14-litre Oxfam buckets, or large plastic drums which were filled up voluntarily, or by the latrine attendants, or through harvesting rainwater from the latrine

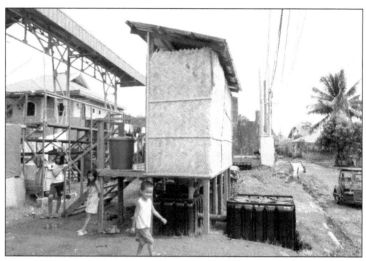

Figure 7.5 Raised latrines in high water table areas © Andy Bastable

rooftops. In an urban setting, as everywhere, the routine and regular filling up of communal hand washing stations is a task that is often neglected. Our quandary is do we continue with communal hand washing devices in urban settings which are often vandalized (for instance by children), or are not routinely filled up, or do we consider providing them exclusively with household devices, or a combination of both (communal and household)?

Community participation and latrine management. From the outset of the response in Haiti, Pakistan, and the Philippines, Oxfam GB ensured that the community participated in the construction of the latrine facilities: for instance in Haiti there were many skilled carpenters and plumbers who were idle and needed a source of income. Their participation also ensured a level of ownership of the facilities.

The three main management models used for the sanitation facilities implemented by Oxfam GB were:

- communal toilets, maintained by volunteers;
- communal toilets, maintained by paid attendants;
- shared family latrines, maintained by 4–5 families on a voluntary basis, and the shared latrines were equipped with a padlock and a set of keys.

At the Petion Ville Golf Course camp a series of WASH activities were undertaken in the camp using paid labourers to clean and maintain community latrines, and to collect and dispose of solid waste in the camp.

Initially, paid community mobilizers were selected by the camp committees and established in five sectors, five people per sector. Early on, 20 people were employed in each camp sector. People were employed for a period of two weeks and then rotated. However, there was dissatisfaction with the selection process for both community mobilizers and waste management staff, including complaints and in some cases protests and threats against Oxfam GB. In response, social events were organized on a regular basis with music, dance, and other activities. A 'lottery' of camp resident names took place during the event, with people being selected randomly. Events not only acted as a psychological support for camp residents, but were successful in reducing tensions amongst the camp population as well.

One key point to consider is the cost/benefit of putting such a system in place. Events are more expensive than traditional community mobilizer selection techniques, but increase overall acceptance.

For the long term, the phasing out of latrine attendants required allocating a number of families to each latrine, and providing them with keys and a padlock to ensure their use and management of the individual latrine.

Manual desludging. Owing to high usage, and limited vehicular access, latrines were desludged manually by the *Bayacoo* (a traditional group that worked only at night). Oxfam GB provided equipment: buckets and rope; safety equipment including boots, overalls, gloves, and facemasks; and cleaning materials including soap and chlorine solution. A dedicated *Bayacoo*-only shower unit was also built for the workers. Prior to undertaking the desludging, *Bayacoo* threw a mix of chlorine solution, disinfectant, and diesel fuel into the pit to 'sterilize' the contents (this is a traditional practice and probably has limited effect).

The plastic buckets were removed from the site by pick-up truck and taken to the only major dumpsite (Truitier) in Haiti for disposal. Plastic buckets with screw lids were used to maximize transport, and prevent any spillages.

Mechanical desludging. Oxfam GB procured two vacuum suction trucks to assist with faecal sludge management in Haiti, and the trucks were donated to DINEPA, the local water/sewerage authority. Oxfam GB also contracted Disaster Waste Recovery (INGO) to assist DINEPA to set up a Vacuum Truck Fleet Management Unit. The project was then handed over to UNOPS. One constraint with this activity was very long delays experienced with customs for the release of the vehicles, which greatly hampered the implementation of the Fleet Management Project.

A number of hand-operated diaphragm sludge pumps were also purchased to assist in desludging latrine pits. The pumps were trialled at the golf course, but were found to be ineffective owing to the high volume of solid waste thrown into the pits. The waste effectively blocked the pump diaphragm; as a result, Oxfam GB employed *Bayacoo* to carry out manual desludging.

Final disposal. Final disposal of faecal matter proved one of the most contentious issues in Haiti, as only one major dumpsite (Truitier) exists. The site is unsuitable environmentally (solid, faecal, and medical waste were deposited in the same vicinity) and poorly managed. However, given the lack of viable alternatives, organizations were forced to discharge faecal sludge at Truitier. One year later, in spite of strong lobbying from the international community, no alternative facilities have been created because of the lack of land. Inaction by agencies and the complex nature of land tenure in Haiti have also been a factor. Disaster Waste Recovery (DWR) designed and implemented a waste stabilization pond, yet near completion it had to be cancelled because of a conflict over land ownership, DWR are now commencing works at a new site, where the land ownership issue has been scrutinized.

Specific to Haiti, communities required that all pit latrines have ventilation pipes installed. Despite explaining the purpose of the ventilation pipes, and the fact that the latrines did not operate as ventilated improved latrines, the ventilation pipes were added as an aesthetic add-on, to make them acceptable by the community.

Women expressed their concerns with the squatting latrine slabs, and attributed vaginal infections to using the latrines (namely the hot air rising from beneath the pit when they opened the keyhole cover). Through women's group discussions, the hygiene promoters had to explain that squatting slabs have been used in many different countries, with similar climates, and no such health condition had prevailed for the female population.

Lessons identified

Lessons learned are notoriously negative, but over the last 2 years, in view of Haiti, Pakistan, and the Philippines, humanitarian agencies have learned a great deal and in a positive way.

- Biodegradable bags are a good feasible option when there is no toilet option and/or in the first couple of weeks in responding to an urban disaster, until regular pit latrines are constructed.
- Urine diversion latrines in emergencies do have a role to play, especially as they reduce the volume of solid matter and mean that the waste is drier and easier to manage and transport. This system, however, does necessitate regular (paid) latrine attendants.
- Painting hygiene promotion murals on the latrines is an effective way to communicate hygiene messages, promoting ownership and use.
- Paid latrine attendants are a short-term measure: the allocation of family latrines with keys and padlocks helps to safeguard use and sustainability in the long term.
- Operation and maintenance of latrines should also include hand washing stations, particularly when these are communal. As with communal latrines, attendants should be paid to ensure water and soap is readily available and stations are cleaned and maintained.
- In an urban context, the Sphere indicators for the number of latrines may not need to apply. In Haiti, camps were equipped with 1 latrine for every 100, or even 150 people. Monitoring of queue times, inflated camp populations, and people going home to their neighbour's toilet, helped us come to the conclusion that number of latrines was flexible, on a case-by-case basis.

Initiatives related to increasing our effectiveness in responding to sanitation in emergencies

For a number of years Oxfam GB has been hosting emergency sanitation forums with a view to improving sanitation in emergencies. The Oxfam slab, which became the Interagency plastic latrine slab, was also a product of these forums. The first of these forums was held in Oxford in 1995. Since this time we have explored new ideas from the development (rather than humanitarian) field and started using CLTS (community-led total sanitation) and urine diversion in emergencies, but still, progress in the sector when compared with progress in the water sector has been minuscule. This year the landscape shows signs of changing; a number of suppliers including the two British companies that provide much of the water equipment have started producing sanitation equipment. There is now more interest from donors, such as DFID, OFDA, and the Dutch Government in emergency sanitation. One hopes that with this upsurge of attention, we can give the sector the huge boost it has been awaiting for the last 30 years.

The last two emergency sanitation forums have been held at Stoutenburg, Netherlands. The outcome of the last meeting was a very clear list of what is still missing in the sanitation sector, in order to promote effective means to respond to sanitation in emergencies.

- better no-toilet options – biodegradable plastic bags;
- squatting latrine slab (cheaper, better alternative to what currently exists);
- urine diversion latrine slab;
- sitting latrine slab;
- latrine slab for smaller people (children);
- latrine slab for less-able people;
- latrine superstructure;
- raised latrine kit;
- latrine lining kits;
- hand desludging pumps;
- mechanical desludging options;
- sludge collection, treatment, and disposal;
- hand washing device.

Items 2–6 can be in the way of ancillaries, that is, add-ons to existing latrine slabs developed.

Many of these equipment-based gaps are currently receiving attention from a few agencies but as yet we have not seen a leap forward in emergency equipment, particularly related to sludge collection, treatment, and disposal. Oxfam GB, with humanitarian equipment specialists such as Nag Magic and Even Products, have already initiated proactive developments in closing the gap in emergency sanitation. Nag Magic has developed ancillaries that can be added to its existing squatting slab, in order to produce a urine diversion latrine slab and Aircell has designed a sitting latrine slab, whereas Even Products has developed a raised latrine and superstructure, and a lining kit.

108 WATER, SANITATION AND HYGIENE IN HUMANITARIAN CONTEXTS

With regard to the hand washing device, a device is needed that can be added to an existing household water container, which will conserve water, allow hands-free hand washing (hands must be free to wash, rather than pour) and will permit an adequate flow of water to lather and wash hands with soap/ash. Again similar to the sanitation equipment, there are a few suppliers working on this initiative.

Recommendations and conclusions

As safe excreta disposal can have such a huge impact on the health of vulnerable people affected by crises it is still shocking that the majority of money goes to water supply often at the expensive of safe sanitation. What is required is for major donors and individual agencies to always advocate not only for adequate safe excreta disposal but also for excreta disposal with dignity. Designs genuinely need to take into account the user's preference and ensure that special accommodation is made for less able people, children, and the elderly after consultation with them.

Is it sufficient just to dig a hole, put a plastic slab on it, dig in four poles, and wrap some plastic sheeting around it? In many cultures women do not like to be seen entering the toilets so at the very least a privacy barrier needs to be erected. In many situations people cut or try to steal the plastic sheeting or the wind rips

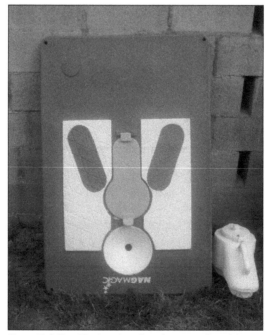

Figure 7.6 Nag Magic urine diversion squatting slab (urine, faeces, and anal cleansing). Right of the slab – children's potty

INNOVATIVE DESIGNS AND APPROACHES IN SANITATION 109

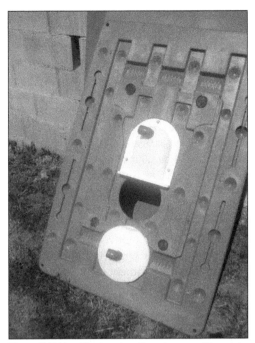

Figure 7.7 Nag Magic urine diversion squatting slab-underside

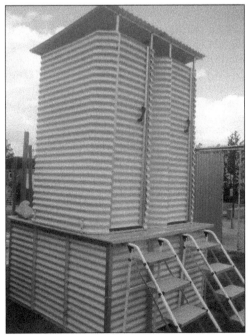

Figure 7.8 Even Products raised latrine and superstructure

it, and while we are often told it is only temporary, the reality is that more often than not they end up being long-term installations. Why not prepare for this in advance and provide better quality toilets which in turn will encourage larger and more sustained use of these facilities? In the long term this will be a much more cost-effective response than some sticks and plastic sheeting.

Agencies also need to think more consistently about how latrines will be desludged before the design stage, bearing in mind that short-term solutions often turn into long-term facilities. The issue of the final deposit site for desludged material is also often overlooked as agencies are not always able to check where the tanker off-loads. We should be taking more responsibility for ensuring that: 1) it gets to the proper site; and 2) that the site does represent a 'safe' disposal site.

About the authors

Andy Bastable is a Public Health Engineering Coordinator with Oxfam GB and **Jenny Lamb** is Public Health Engineering Advisor for HECA and West Africa within the Humanitarian Department of Oxfam.

References

Fewtrell, L., Kaufmann, R.B., Kay, D., Enanoria, W., Haller, L. and Colford, J.M. Jr (2005) 'Water, sanitation, and hygiene interventions to reduce diarrhoea in less developed countries: A systematic review and meta-analysis'. Lancet Infectious Diseases 5:42–52, http://dx.doi.org/10.1016/S1473-3099(04)01253-8

JMP (2008) *Estimates for the use of improved drinking-water sources and improved sanitation facilities,* WHO/UNICEF Joint Monitoring Programme for Water Supply and Sanitation, Geneva, updated March 2010.

Oxfam GB *Technical Brief 2 Vulnerability and Socio-cultural Considerations for PHE in Emergencies* [website], Oxfam GB <http://www.oxfam.org.uk/resources/downloads/emerg_manuals/draft_oxfam_tech_brief_sociocultural.pdf> [accessed 22 November 2011].

Oxfam GB (2010a) *Technical Brief 19: The Use of Poo Bags for Safe Excreta Disposal in Emergency Settings* [website], Oxfam GB <http://policy-practice.oxfam.org.uk/publications/the-use-of-poo-bags-for-safe-excreta-disposal-in-emergency-settings-136535> [accessed 22 November 2011].

Oxfam GB (2010b) 'Enquête sur les moyens d'existence et le marché local de l'eau dans l'aire métropolitaine de Port-au-Prince', http://www.pseau.org/outils/ouvrages/oxfam_enquete_marche_de_leau_port_au_prince_haiti_fr.pdf

Oxfam GB (2011) *Technical Brief 20: Urban WASH Lessons Learned from Post-Earthquake Response in Haiti* [website], Oxfam GB <http://policy-practice.oxfam.org.uk/publications/urban-wash-lessons-learned-from-post-earthquake-response-in-haiti-136538> [accessed 22 November 2011].

Oxfam International (2011a) *Haiti Progress Report 2010* [website], Oxfam International <http://www.oxfam.org/en/policy/haiti-progress-report-2010> [accessed 22 November 2011].

Oxfam International (2011b) 'From relief to recovery: Supporting good governance in post-earthquake Haiti', *Oxfam Briefing Paper* 142 [website], Oxfam International <http://www.oxfam.org/en/policy/relief-recovery> [accessed 22 November 2011].

Patel, D., Brooks, N. and Bastable, A. (2011) 'Excreta disposal in emergencies: Bag and Peepoo trials with internally displaced people in Port-au-Prince', http://dx.doi.org/10.3362/1756-3488.2011.006.

CHAPTER 8

Biodegradable bags as emergency sanitation in urban settings: the field experience

Francesca Coloni, Rafael van den Bergh, Federico Sittaro, Stephanie Giandonato, Geneviève Loots and Peter Maes

Abstract

In addition to the dire medical needs resulting from the 2010 Haiti earthquake, over 1.5 million people were left without access to sanitation facilities. In the second phase of the overall emergency response, Médecins Sans Frontières-Operational Centre Brussels attempted to address the urgent need for safe and sanitary human excreta disposal in some of the most neglected camps for displaced people in Port-au-Prince, by implementing an approach consisting of defecation in single-use, biodegradable plastic bags. Construction and maintenance of facilities for this intervention was undemanding and cost-effective, and the approach offered a suitable solution to a number of technical constraints encountered in this urban setting. However, immediate acquisition of ecologically appropriate bags proved troublesome. Furthermore, a relatively low bag usage rate of 13 per cent (8–18 per cent) was observed, differing considerably from the rates reported in more controlled evaluations of such approaches, reflecting the operational limitations to this intervention. We therefore recommend this sanitation approach in urban settings only as a stop-gap approach when other interventions are not possible.

Keywords: humanitarian sanitation, pit latrines, biodegradable bags, environmental burden

In the wake of the 12 January 2010 earthquake that struck Port-au-Prince, Haiti, at least 1,500,000 people (UN OCHA, 2010) were left without a home, social infrastructure, or adequate access to sanitation facilities. The scale of the disaster and its consequences placed an exceptional burden on the already poor country and introduction of sanitary practices for the displaced population proved to be a major challenge. By March 2010, two months after the earthquake, toilets were only available for 1 in 400 persons, falling well short of the ratio of 1 per 100 persons targeted by the inter-agency emergency Water, Hygiene, and Sanitation (WASH) Cluster and its implementing partners (WASH, 2010) – itself only 20 per cent of the Sphere minimum standard of 1 per 20 (The Sphere Project,

2004). Even after four months (May 2010), the ratio of latrines per person was approximately 1 in 190, and in June 2010 a household survey on water, sanitation, and hygiene conducted by the Centers for Disease Control (CDC) in internally displaced people (IDP) camps, indicated that only 66.2 per cent of the respondents used a latrine in or in the immediate vicinity of the camps (CDC, 2010). Furthermore, 7.2 per cent reported using a canal or other open area for defecation. Such a lack of sanitation facilities for a prolonged period of time in such circumstances constitutes a clear and present public health threat. In addition, it can increase the strong feeling of a lack of dignity for a population already heavily affected by a disaster such as the Haiti earthquake.

Constraints to implementation of sanitation measures

A number of constraints specific to the Haiti/Port-au-Prince post-earthquake setting impeded a rapid implementation of sanitary measures, in particular for human excreta disposal. The first clear complication was the densely constructed fabric of the city where collapsed buildings were still taking a lot of space. The areas spontaneously occupied by the population for their settlement were on average highly overpopulated. Apart from shelters there was very little remaining space to devote to infrastructures such as toilets, bathing facilities, etc.

Secondly, the uncertainty over the final locations of the IDP camps and the population effectively residing in them complicated the identification of a proper place and a correct number of toilets for each settlement, precluding the proper planning of a sanitation strategy. In particular, the population size within the settlements was difficult to estimate owing to: resistance from the population to move into the officially recognized camps out of fear they would develop into shanty towns; security threats forcing people to search for other refuges; use of the camps at night only; creation of fake encampments – the so-called 'ghost camps' – to attract humanitarian aid; and evacuation of camps in flood-prone areas during the rainy season.

Other challenges pertaining to sanitation efforts were at a more practical level. The high water table, rocky soil close to the surface, or the fact that camps were installed in the middle of the urban context on impermeable terrains (squares, parking lots, tarred surfaces) or in locations where the owners did not allow the digging of pits (football fields, golf courses), necessitated the use of either elevated toilets connected to a reservoir (a relatively resource-consuming approach) or of portable ones.

Desludging capacity was particularly limited in the aftermath of the disaster: only a few private trucks were providing an unreliable and very expensive service. In the case of portable toilets, the cost was up to US$20/cabin/day (including both rent and daily emptying). Additionally, the official landfill had a very limited reception capacity, being overwhelmed by the dumping of different types of waste produced in Port-au-Prince (from medical waste and debris from destroyed buildings up to the waste generated by the huge international community temporarily living in Port-Au-Prince).

Aims

In this complex environment, the capacity of many actors to intervene efficiently was quickly overstretched, resulting in gaps and delays from which it was difficult to recover. Innovative approaches to providing adequate sanitation were therefore urgently needed. Most agencies involved in WASH activities focused on the implementation of techniques such as simple, ventilated, and raised pits. To answer the dire need for rapid control of indiscriminate defecation by initiation of temporary measures (which could be improved later on), we opted to implement a rapid approach consisting of defecation in single-use, biodegradable plastic bags. A similar concept was also explored in Haiti by Patel et al. (2011) in a formal trial under relatively controlled conditions; here, we present our operational field experience as a counterpart to this documented trial.

Methodology

Human excreta disposal: Conceptual approach

Initially, Médecins Sans Frontières-Operational Centre Brussels (MSF-OCB) focused its emergency response to the earthquake on provision of medical care, including an important surgical component (Chu et al., 2011). As the overall needs of many people in the IDP camps were still unmet by March 2010 and in particular in areas neglected because of the precarious security situation (e.g. Cité Soleil, Sarthe), MSF-OCB provided 'package assistance' to 15 camps and 22,765 persons through distribution of tents, non-food item kits, sanitation, and hygiene promotion activities. Specifically in the context of sanitation, a first response consisting of a temporary sanitation method was deemed appropriate, considering the precarious living conditions of the population.

Based on these considerations and the constraints discussed above, we opted for a phased approach. In the initial phase, an existing practice in Haiti – defecation in single-use plastic bags – was adapted and adopted as a stop-gap measure. Specific adaptations included the rapid introduction of biodegradable plastic bags, the construction of temporary community cubicles and the organized collection of used bags for proper disposal, to counter the 'flying toilet' custom (UNDP, 2006). A second phase would then consist of the replacement of these temporary toilets with more permanent ones (ventilated, raised, or with buried tanks).

Toilet construction: Methods and materials

For the implementation of the first phase, a carpentry shop consisting of 15 workers and an 'installation team' consisting of four technicians were organized, and a number of cubicle prototypes were tested.

Separate cubicles for male and female use were constructed. For the calculation of the required number of cubicles, it was assumed that one cubicle could serve between 100 and 150 persons as the accumulation rate is not an issue with this type of toilet. In the camps the identification of the toilet sites was done in consultation with the community. The installation procedure comprised preparation of the terrain, gravel layering, covering of the floor with plastic sheeting, mounting of the cubicles and fencing off of the area.

Three different types of bag were used. All had the same size and design – approximately 10 litre capacity, T-shirt shape with two handles, dark coloured, not transparent – but differed in material and supplier (Table 8.1). For the initial trial period, ordinary plastic bags were purchased locally. For the scale-up, biodegradable bags were purchased in Santo Domingo and – when these turned out to be incompliant with EN 13432:2000 norms – in Europe.

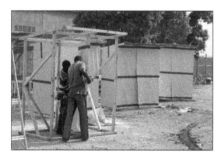 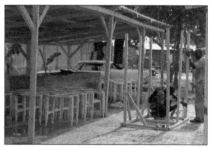

Figure 8.1 The cubicles are constructed

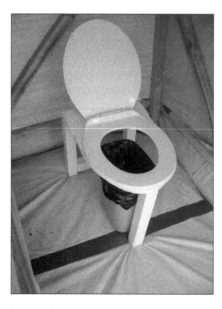 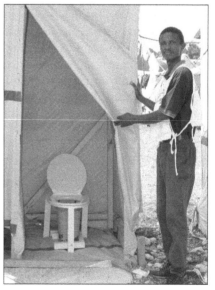

Figure 8.2 The completed cubicles

Table 8.1 Specifics on the bags used

	Type 1	Type 2	Type 3
Ecological properties biodegradable	Biofragmentable	Allegedly	Biodegradable
EN 13432:2000 compliant	No	No	Yes
Provenance	Haiti	Santo Domingo	Europe
Size (cm × cm)	35 × 40	41 × 46	30 × 35
Cost (€cent/pc)	0.7	9.8	6 (without transport)
Quantity ordered (pcs)	60,000	40,000	100,000

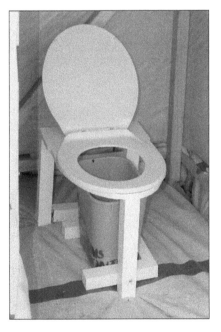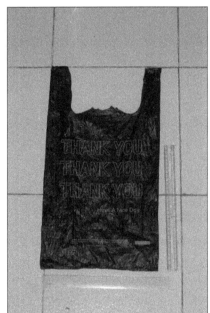

Figure 8.3 The pee-poo bag, and how it is disposed

To ensure proper use and correct bag disposal, distribution was centralized at the cubicle level. The hygiene committee of each camp appointed attendants (1 per 10 toilets) who had the multiple tasks of supervising the toilets, explaining their use, distributing the bags, and cleaning. Outside, covered plastic bins of 60 litre capacity, one per five cubicles, were installed for the disposal of used bags. These bins were collected to be emptied in the final disposal site (the landfill of Port-au-Prince) and replaced with cleaned and disinfected ones; collection was done daily, except in a small number of camps where collection was only possible 2–3 times per week.

Bag consumption was foreseen as 4 bags/woman/day (i.e. for collection of faeces and urine) and 1 bag/man/day (i.e. for collection of faeces only). In total, 191,200 bags were distributed.

Timeline of the intervention

Use of these toilets started at the beginning of April (week 14). The intervention was foreseen to last 2 months (i.e. 8 weeks), allowing the time both to understand which camps would stay longer and to prepare for the second phase of the approach relying on two desludging trailers which were at that point en route to Haiti.

In reality, toilets were used for different lengths of time. The temporary setup finally lasted till the end of September, reflecting the operational constraints to implementing the second phase in a timely manner. Acquisition of distribution and collection data was maintained till the end of July (week 29) for a total of 4 months (i.e. 16 weeks).

Data collection

Data analysis was based only on routine supply and waste processing data, no data on human subjects was collected or analysed in this study. Approach evaluation was based mainly on the personal appreciation and experiences of the hygiene promotion personnel involved in the construction and maintenance of the toilets.

Results and discussion

Appreciation of the practical aspects of the intervention

At the technical level, the intervention was evaluated positively. Specific benefits of the approach included its rapid implementation: the workshop and installation teams managed to produce and install 16 toilets/day because of the low material requirements, the simple standard design, and the easy installation (no digging required). The high mobility of the toilets was particularly advantageous in following the movements of the population, e.g. after flooding necessitated the evacuation of certain camps. Additionally, the size of the cubicle (0.64 m^2) was considerably smaller than the recommended size of a traditional toilet (0.96 m^2), indicating that three biodegradable plastic bag toilet cubicles (serving 300 persons) can be accommodated in an area for only two traditional toilets (serving 40 persons) (Reed, 2010). Environmental contamination was minimized thanks to the storage and transport of excreta in closed bags and covered collection bins. No detectable pollution of nearby water sources and reservoirs, either ground or surface, was caused at the location of the toilet. However, the system did result in an environmental burden at the final disposal site of the bags, as the sludge remained untreated.

This is particularly problematic in a context such as Port-au-Prince, where only one landfill services the entire city of more than 2 million inhabitants (UN OCHA, 2010).

At the maintenance and usage level, too, several positive aspects were noted. Regular cleaning was sufficient as general maintenance and the collection of full bins using simple trucks circumvented the need for desludging. Different levels of hygiene promotion activity were required. On the one hand, demands for actual explanation of the use of the toilets were limited, as the use of plastic bags for defecation was already widely adopted by the population. Consequently, a balance needed to be found between formal compulsory explanatory hygiene promotion sessions and rapid deployment of the structures. On the other hand, the management of the entire sanitation approach was demanding and could have benefited from a more structured presence of a hygiene team. Maintaining the system of cleaning and monitoring and distribution on a voluntary basis was a particular challenge in this context.

At the technical level, bag capacity was enough to contain both urine/faeces and provided material for personal cleansing. Bags proved to be resistant enough for their purposes – transfer operations did not result in spillage of excreta. No problem of leakages in the outside collection bucket were reported. Additionally, despite initial fears, formation of high amounts of biogas causing tightened bags to explode was not reported.

Several issues were encountered with the purchasing of the disposable bags. The first batch, purchased locally, was biofragmentable only, and was sufficient for the initial launching of the project and evaluation of appreciation by the population. The second batch, purchased in Santo Domingo, was more expensive and turned out to be only biofragmentable, too, rather than biodegradable, resulting in some environmental pollution. The third batch consisted of biodegradable bags ordered in Europe that took a long time to be produced (because of their short shelf-life suppliers keep a very limited ready-to-ship stock) and had a high price tag (Table 8.1) in addition to the transport costs.

Monitoring of the approach

Over the course of the intervention, a total of 15 camps were provided with a total of 197 toilet cubicles for the use of plastic bags. On a weekly basis, on average 119 toilets were in use, ranging from 49 to 165. Over all the IDP camps, a relatively low average bag usage rate of 13 per cent (ranging from 8 to 18 per cent) was observed. This rate differed significantly from the high usage rates identified in the Peepoo® trial documented by Patel et al. (2011). On the one hand, this may be explained by over-estimation of the IDP population living in the camps (camp only inhabited at night, shift to other sanitation facilities in the vicinity during the intervention, etc.), or by a general lower appreciation of the approach by the population – community cubicles only versus community cubicles and household use in the Peepoo® trial. On the

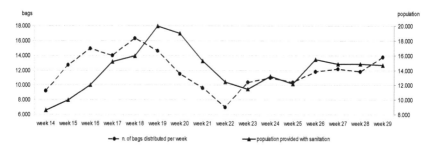

Figure 8.1 Plastic bag distribution versus population

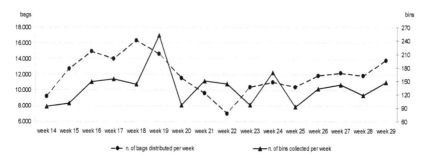

Figure 8.2 Plastic bag distribution versus outside collection bins collected

other hand, this discrepancy may reflect the inherent differences between a small-scale trial in controlled settings (4,060 Peepoo® bags plus an unspecified number of biofragmentable plastic bags distributed, covering 2,211 persons over a total period of 6 weeks) and the operational reality of a full-scale intervention in the field (191,200 bags distributed to 22,765 persons over 4 months).

In general, the number of distributed bags tended to follow the size of the population receiving sanitation care (Figure 8.1) and the number of collected bins (Figure 8.2), reflecting the consistency in their usage rates. Several phenomena lay at the root of the decreasing trend during weeks 19–22 and the sharply decreased bin collection in week 25, including unexpected logistical constraints (such as the breakdown in week 20 of the truck in charge of bin collection and the destruction of two camps by a hurricane), a reduced presence in two camps due to specific security restrictions, and a delay in receiving the biodegradable plastic bags, forcing a slowing down of the programme.

Recommendations and ways forward

Several recommendations can be formulated from this experience. The implementation of single-use biodegradable plastic bag toilets in an urban post-earthquake intervention was recognized a posteriori as an efficient immediate response (Reed, 2010). Additionally, the system seems compatible with other emergency scenarios, such as floods and hurricanes/cyclones in urban contexts, or in IDP/refugee camps. We therefore consider it to be an adequate stop-gap approach to be used when other, more elaborate interventions are not applicable. However, there are several caveats:

1. Use of biodegradable material is a requisite to keep the environmental burden to a minimum and – as was the case in Haiti – such materials are not necessarily readily available immediately post-catastrophe. An emergency preparedness stock of such bags could be provided, though this would have to be reconciled with the relatively short shelf-life of such bags.
2. The site of final disposal should be well-considered, as the faecal matter itself is not treated in any way.
3. Institutionalization of temporary measures should be avoided; in the case of the intervention described here, temporary toilets were still in use after 4 months, despite the intention to phase-out after 2 months.
4. The system should be strongly discouraged during outbreaks of faecal-oral transmissible diseases (diarrhoea/cholera) because of the high risk of contamination linked with the direct manipulation of the bags.

Overall, the authors recommend that the implementation of such a sanitation methodology is repeated in other countries and the results analysed, in order to confirm whether biodegradable plastic bag toilets are a valid option to be considered more often in emergency responses. Results could, for instance, significantly differ in settings where defecation in plastic bags is not an established practice. Specific improvements could be incorporated in future interventions:

1. Self-sanitising bags, such as the Peepoo® bags in the trial documented by Patel et al. (2011), which disinfect the contents, prevent biogas formation, and reduce the odour, could be used, on the condition that they are extremely easy in use, their timely delivery or shelf-life are suitable for emergency response purposes, and pricing is acceptable.
2. Implementation at the household level in addition to the community approach could significantly reduce the feelings of insecurity and lack of privacy in the IDP camps. Additionally, it would have allowed access to sanitation facilities at night. An operational research study aimed specifically at the difference in acceptance between household- and community-level intervention could be designed.
3. Full exploitation of the modular design of the intervention should be considered: the superstructure initially used as cubicles for single-use bags could have been prepared for reinstallation in the second phase as part of more traditional (e.g. simple, ventilated, and raised pits) toilets.
4. The use of bags only for faeces could be implemented, while an integrated urine-diversion system for liquids provides a real 'full package' sanitation service.

    5. Closer involvement of the local authorities should be envisaged; in this intervention, information was only shared on the Cluster platform, and local authorities were not bilaterally contacted.

Acknowledgements

The authors would like to thank Patrick Tavernier for his initiative in the early stages of the intervention.

About the authors

Francesca Coloni, Federico Sittaro, and **Stephanie Giandonato** are with Médecins Sans Frontières, Operations Department, **Brussels,** and **Rafael Van den Bergh** (Rafael.VAN.DEN.BERGH@brussels.msf.org), **Geneviève Loots**, and **Peter Maes** are with Médecins Sans Frontières, Medical Department, Brussels, Belgium.

References

CDC (2010) *Access to Water, Sanitation and Hygiene In IDP Settlements in Port-au-Prince, Haiti, Results of a Household Survey (conducted in June 2010)*, CDC, Atlanta, Draft 4 August 2010.

Chu, K., Stokes, C., Trelles, M. and Ford, N. (2011) 'Improving effective surgical delivery in humanitarian disasters: Lessons from Haiti', *PLoS Med* 8: e1001025.

Patel, D., Brooks, N. and Bastable, A. (2011) 'Excreta disposal in emergencies: Bag and Peepoo trials with internally displaced people in Port-au-Prince', *Waterlines* 30: 62–77.

Reed, W. (2010) *Emergency Excreta Disposal Standards and Options for Haiti*, WEDC, Leicestershire, UK.

Sphere Project (2004) *Humanitarian Charter and Minimum Standards in Humanitarian Response* [website], Oxfam GB, Oxford <http://www.sphereproject.org/> [last accessed 30 January 2012].

UN OCHA (2010) 'Key Facts and Figures', internal document, UN OCHA, New York.

UNDP (2006) *Human Development Report. Beyond Scarcity: Power, Poverty and the Global Water Crisis*, UNDP, New York.

WASH (2010) 'WASH Cluster Sanitation Strategy for Going to Scale', final draft 7 March 2010 <http://www.redr.org.uk/washmaterials/content/S%20-%20WASH%20Strategy/S1%20-%20Introduction/S1_HO_Haiti%20Sanitation%20strategy.pdf> [last accessed 1 February 2012].

CHAPTER 9
Urban armed conflicts and water services

Jean-François Pinera

Abstract

Many of the recent armed conflicts have affected cities of the developing world. In the resulting emergency situations, water supply is among the most essential services to restore. It forms part of urban services commonly managed by local water sector institutions. This article is based on case-study research carried out in six war-afflicted cities and towns that looked at how partnerships between aid agencies and water sector institutions influenced aid operations benefits. In emergency operations, findings showed that partnerships did not necessarily influence the efficiency or effectiveness of the response in the short term but were beneficial because they prepared for rehabilitation. During rehabilitation, findings suggested that current practice maintains a separation between large-scale rehabilitation projects and community-based projects focusing on specific neighbourhoods. This has a detrimental effect on sustainability and fails to address the needs of the most vulnerable populations. The research recommended a more coordinated approach in order to reconcile sustainability and universal service.

Keywords: armed conflicts; humanitarian relief; urban areas; water and sanitation

Developing countries are becoming increasingly urban. According to the United Nations Population Division (2009), urban populations in the less developed regions will be larger than rural populations by 2020. In addition, developing countries are prone to social unrest, which in the worst of its manifestations may turn into armed conflicts. The vast majority of armed conflicts that have erupted since 1946 took place in developing countries (Themnér and Wallensteen, 2011). It is therefore hardly surprising that as many as 150 cities and towns from developing countries have been affected by armed conflicts between 1975 and 2004 (Pinera and Reed, 2007: 403). One of the main reasons explaining this trend is that cities are usually considered as decisive targets by rebels who see them as symbols of power and wealth. Moreover, in cities, unemployed male youth can easily be recruited as fighters (Murshed, 2002: 389).

The provision of essential services to city dwellers requires relatively complex infrastructure. Targeting this infrastructure during armed conflicts has been a common occurrence, either as a result of collateral or unintended damage or as a strategy to weaken opponents and prevent resources from being diverted from war (Anand, 2005: 2). Water supply is among the services that are frequently targeted. This applies to water infrastructure, which may be damaged or destroyed, as well as to the institutions in charge of running the service, which may lose personnel and assets.

The consequences of urban armed conflicts on water supply are considerable human suffering and may prompt the intervention of the so-called 'international community' in order to help restore a minimum level of service. In doing so, aid agencies involved are confronted with complex situations, in which the relationship between consumers and service providers has changed. When the latter have disappeared or are incapacitated, agencies may substitute them. A return to 'normal' should then depend on repair or reconstruction of the damaged infrastructure. However, this is only the tip of the iceberg. Long-lasting crises have an 'eroding effect' on institutions and societies (Duffield, 1994: 38), which makes problems persistent beyond the mere reconstruction process. In order to take into account this longer perspective, it is essential that aid agencies deal both with social and institutional aspects of assistance. This implies, in particular, interacting with water sector institutions.

The mechanisms of such interaction were the object of a study of how the partnerships between aid agencies and water sector institutions influence the outcome of emergency response and rehabilitation projects. It was carried out by the author at Loughborough University (United Kingdom) between 2004 and 2006. This article summarizes its main findings and conclusions.

The research

Justification and aim

The research emerged from the author's practical experience of working in urban areas affected by armed conflicts (especially Kabul), where aid workers often consider dealing with local institutions as a problem. This is mostly due to the contradiction between a declared intention by aid agencies to work with longer-term objectives and aid strategies, which do not give them the means to achieve this ambition. Both aid agencies and donors defend the 'relief to development link' (Buchanan-Smith and Maxwell, 1994), which means consolidating local capacities in order to ensure longer-terms benefits of relief. Yet in practice, and especially when local capacities depend on local government, difficulties often appear.

During acute emergencies, aid agencies may neglect institutions because they see them as not sufficiently efficient to deliver quick results. When rehabilitation or reconstruction is carried out, local institutions may be considered as unacceptable or unsuitable partners. This is often due to political concerns or to institutions being regarded as too inefficient and/or corrupt.

In some cases, these concerns may be legitimate; however, this reflects a general 'state avoidance' tendency which has been a characteristic of the work of most relief agencies in recent years (Slaymaker et al., 2005: 32). Whilst some aspects of the problem are perceived as inherent in local institutions, others are purely the result of characteristics of aid agencies and aid policy. Firstly, working in partnership with local institutions in cities affected by armed conflicts requires carrying out tasks such as institutional development, which are not appealing to most aid agencies (Smillie, 2001: 20) because they usually lack the competence to do so. Secondly, supporting local institutions entails a commitment over relatively long periods, which is something hardly compatible with most funding patterns.

The research aimed at finding out how these partnerships may nonetheless take place in order to maximize aid benefits. Emergency response and rehabilitation were considered separately.

Methodology

The parameters considered to estimate aid benefits were efficiency and effectiveness, which are preponderant in the case of emergency operations, in addition to sustainability, and coverage. They are defined as follows:

- Determining efficiency and effectiveness consists of an input/output analysis. Efficiency compares the benefits of the intervention for each target group over the considered period with the resources mobilized. These resources may be: equipment, consumables, manpower, expertise, and cash. Effectiveness compares what was set as an objective with what was actually achieved.
- Evaluating sustainability entails defining what elements are threats to the continuity of benefits from the considered response and whether the recipient population/institution is able to overcome these threats.
- Coverage estimates the proportion of the target population that benefits from assistance. At the level of a city or town, it may also be seen as the proportion of its entire population that is covered. This parameter is particularly important when looking at whether aid operations benefit low-income communities.

The selected methodology was multi-case study research, using specific emergency operation or rehabilitation projects in determined urban areas as unit of analysis (i.e. the nature of the case). For convenience, they are designated as 'interventions'.

For each intervention, the way in which water sector institutions and aid agencies interacted was analysed and conclusions drawn on how the nature and level of partnership between water sector institutions and aid agencies related to aid benefits.

Cases were selected from amongst the armed conflicts that have affected developing countries in the decade previous to the research. They covered six cities and towns, representing a wide range of situations and geographical areas. Data and empirical evidence were based predominantly upon reports, field visits and interviews with expatriate and national staff from aid agencies, staff from water sector institutions, and members of the recipient population.

Areas and agencies

The selection of cases aimed at providing a sufficiently wide range of armed conflict situations in different environments in terms of location and size of the urban centres. They are listed in Table 9.1.

Table 9.1 Countries, urban areas, and agencies involved

#	Countries (or territory) and urban areas selected (Population data source: Brinkhoff, 2011)	Agencies involved in emergency response	Agencies involved in rehabilitation
1	Afghanistan: Kabul (about 2.9 million people in 2009)	International NGOs CARE; Solidarités	International NGOs Action Contre la Faim (ACF) International organizations The International Committee of the Red Cross (ICRC)/The Spanish Red Cross Society International financial institutions (IFIs) The German Development Bank: Kreditanstalt für Wiederaufbau (KfW); World Bank
2	Sri Lanka: Jaffna (about 78,000 people in 2007)	International organizations The German Technical Cooperation agency: (GTZ) now the GIZ Deutsche Gesellschaft für Internationale Zusam-menarbeit: the German International Cooperation Agency	International organizations GTZ
3	Liberia: Monrovia (more than 1 million people in 2008)	International NGOs Médecins Sans Frontières (MSF) – Belgium International Organizations GTZ; ICRC; United Nations Children Fund (UNICEF)	International NGOs Oxfam International organizations UNICEF International financial institutions (IFIs) European Union
4	Democratic Republic of Congo: Béni (about 81,000 people in 2004)		International NGOs Solidarités; Aquassistance
5	Haiti: Port-au-Prince (about 2.3 million people in 2009)	International organization ICRC	International NGO Groupe de Recherche et d'Echange Technologique (GRET)
6	Chechnya: Grozny (about 270,000 people in 2010)	International NGOs MSF-Belgium, Merlin International Organizations ICRC	

Historical background

The 1990s saw an increase in the number of armed conflicts. The six countries in which the case studies were selected illustrate this trend:

- Kabul, the capital of Afghanistan, came under heavy fighting between 1992 and 1996 when different *Mujaheddin* (fighter of the holy war) factions struggled for power before being disbanded by the Taliban. They were in turn defeated in 2001 after a short military campaign led by the United States.
- During the same period, war was raging in Sri Lanka between the government and the 'Liberation Tigers of Tamil Eelam' (LTTE) around the Jaffna peninsula, at the northern tip of the island. Jaffna city came under heavy fighting three times between 1986 and 2001.
- In Liberia, war started in 1992 between the government and different rebel factions including Charles Taylor's. In 1997, Taylor became president but another struggle soon started which eventually would lead to his fall in 2003.
- In the eastern region of the Democratic Republic of Congo, war started in 1996 with the rebellion of the Banyamulenge, an ethnic group of the Kivu region. The subsequent war would end with Mobutu's regime. From 1999, the war opposing two ethnic groups of the Ituri region bordering Kivu to the north also affected the area.
- Haiti has been affected by civil unrest ever since the fall of the Duvalier regime in 1986. A military coup in 1991 and intense political repression prompted two external military interventions in 1994 and 2004. There were riots in the capital Port-au-Prince and in the main cities, especially in 2003.
- Finally, war in Chechnya erupted at the end of 1994; three years after the breakaway republic declared its independence from the Russian Federation. Grozny, its capital, was heavily bombed and, by 1996, after a lull that lasted four years, war restarted by the end of 1999 and Russia managed to re-impose its authority while Grozny was again bombed.

Emergency response

Review of the case studies

Emergency response interventions are summarized Table 9.2.

Kabul. Kabul water network was heavily damaged and water distribution was almost totally interrupted between 1992 and 1996. CARE intervened on one of the main well-fields of the city over a period of six months in 1995. The organization repaired and replaced parts of the submersible pumps, surface equipment, and generators that were looted during the fighting. The operation

Table 9.2 Summary of the main emergency operations reviewed

#	Agencies/utilities involved (The name of some of these utilities may have changed since)	Interventions	Period
1	Kabul: CARE, Solidarités/Central Authority for Water Supply and Sewerage (CAWSS)	Repairs and operation of pumping stations and water schemes	1994–1998
2	Jaffna: GTZ/Jaffna Municipal Council (JMC) water services	Water trucking	1996–1997
3	Monrovia: MSF-Belgium, UNICEF, GTZ, ICRC/Liberia Water and Sewerage Corporation (LWSC) – Liberia Electricity Corporation (LEC)	Repairs and operation of power supply and water treatment plants Drilling of two new boreholes	1990–1996
4	Port-au-Prince: ICRC/Centrale Autonome métropolitaine d'Eau Potable (CAMEP)	Repair of two boreholes Repair of tap-stands	12/2004–2005
5	Grozny: MSF-Belgium, ICRC, Merlin/Vodacanal (VDC)	Water trucking Emergency water storage and distribution Repairs on the water distribution network	1995–2006

and maintenance of the well-field was eventually taken over by Solidarités as part of a larger emergency project whose aim was to repair and run 27 water schemes and drill more than 1,000 boreholes equipped with hand-pumps throughout the city. Both Care and Solidarités worked largely independently from CAWSS, which at the time was very weak and fully controlled by the Taliban authorities (Solidarités, 1998).

Jaffna. Bombs and trenches dug during street fighting inflicted considerable damage on Jaffna's water distribution network. As a result, people could only rely on their wells for water supply. The situation was made even worse by water scarcity, which is a characteristic of the Jaffna peninsula. In 1996 and 1997, GTZ (now GIZ) supported JMC water services in their efforts to distribute water to public buildings where displaced people had taken shelter. By April 1997, water reservoirs supplied with tankers were installed in the most crowded areas of the town (van Horen, 2002: 121).

Monrovia. Monrovia was attacked three times during the Liberian civil war. In 1990, rebels damaged beyond repair the dam providing hydro-electric power to the city's water treatment plant. The plant itself and essential parts of the water network were later looted several times.

MSF Belgium, in collaboration with UNICEF, intervened in late 1990 and early 1991 by helping LEC and LWSC set up emergency power supply to the water treatment plant, and thereby restoring a minimum level of water supply in the city. Between March and October 1991 the ICRC took over from UNICEF.

In October 1992, the water treatment plant was attacked and water supply again interrupted. This time water had to be distributed with tankers. The operation involved LWSC, UNICEF, MSF Belgium, and the ICRC. In 1993, GTZ supported the drilling of two boreholes in the south-east of the city in order to supply water tankers operating in the area. GTZ also supported the rehabilitation of the water treatment plant, which eventually led to certain areas of the city being again supplied by the water treatment plant. Areas not reached continued receiving water from tankers (Ockelford, 1993).

Port-au-Prince. Port-au-Prince water infrastructure degradation was mostly due to a lack of maintenance. In addition, constant worsening of living conditions in the countryside caused a large-scale migration to the capital, most migrants ending up in shantytowns, which in 2004 were home to about 800,000 people (Matthieussent and Carlier, 2004). This considerable expansion of low-income areas in Port-au-Prince was accompanied by the development of criminal gangs, especially in the largest one, Cité Soleil, which became a 'no-go zone' for most aid agencies. As a result, the water scheme supplying the area was partly dismantled and ceased functioning. From December 2004, the ICRC launched the rehabilitation of water and sanitation systems in Cité Soleil. It consisted of the rehabilitation of two boreholes and a number of tap-stands, thereby increasing water supply availability. At the same time the organization supported the creation of water committees recognized by the water utility, CAMEP. CAMEP's technicians carried out the whole operation. They were escorted into Cité Soleil by the Haitian Red Cross and the ICRC (ICRC, 2006).

Grozny. Following the destruction of Grozny power plants most water supply sources were interrupted. In February 1995, the ICRC and MSF-Belgium started water distribution from the only water source available which was reaching the city by gravity. Water was collected in an emergency storage facility run by the ICRC. A large number of water distribution points were set up. They were supplied by trucks rented by both organizations. From March 1995, Merlin joined them (Hodgson and Oppliger, 1998). This continued until 2006 albeit at a smaller scale and with interruptions due to fighting. Some of the aid agencies involved changed but the ICRC kept on running the water storage facility throughout the period. Private trucks distributed water to be sold to the general public, while aid agencies supplied institutions (mostly hospitals and orphanages). In addition to water distribution, the ICRC supported the water utility GVC with spare-parts and tools while Merlin's assistance focused on the repair of water pipelines.

Findings

In each of the emergency response situations described above, the results are evaluated in terms of the efficiency and effectiveness of intervention.

In Kabul, where Care and Solidarités carried out emergency repairs with little input from CAWSS, aid agencies contributed to an increase in the amount of clean water available to the recipient community and thus limited the risk of disease spreading.

The same could be said of emergency response in Jaffna, Monrovia, Port au-Prince, and Grozny, where aid agencies involved worked closely with the water utility. In Jaffna, JMC helped with water trucking; in Monrovia, LWSC technicians fixed the water treatment plant; in Port-au-Prince, CAMEP fixed boreholes in Cité Soleil, and in Grozny, GVC helped with 'quick fixes' on the water network.

It would be easy to assume at the outset that levels of partnership may have little influence on the improvement of access to water services. In Kabul, where CARE and Solidarités had a free hand in managing their interventions, efficiency may even have been greater as they could select the most competent personnel available on the market, without being obliged to work with utilities' staff, thus avoiding delays involved in training and procedures. Based on these results, it can be concluded that aid agencies may, during a certain time, substitute local water institutions without detrimental effects and even sometimes with greater benefits. Partnerships are then indispensable only when the complexity of water systems requires the expertise of utilities' staff.

This, however, only considers the short-term timeframe of emergency operations. If effects are considered in the longer term, it is evident that the level of partnership may influence how emergency interventions may be linked to rehabilitation/reconstruction and development. Water sector institutions involved in emergency responses are often also involved in rehabilitation projects and therefore collaboration in the emergency response phase can be seen as the initial step towards a closer relationship between local institutions and international aid. This contributes to prepare and facilitate implementation of rehabilitation and represents a first step in strengthening the capacity of water sector institutions, giving them more credibility with their consumers.

Rehabilitation

Review of the case studies

Rehabilitation response interventions are summarized in Table 9.3.

Kabul. After the fall of the Taliban, KfW and later the World Bank, through the German consulting firm Beller-Kocks, became involved both in capacity building of CAWSS and in the rehabilitation of the water distribution network. It was carried out in two phases: During Phase I, implemented between 2002 and 2004, repairs on the water distribution network were undertaken and assistance delivered to CAWSS in terms of equipment, consumables, vehicles, and training. Phase II, initiated in 2005, provided for the extension of the water distribution network. It was meant to be completed by 2009; however by August 2011 works were very advanced but still ongoing. In addition to

Table 9.3 Summary of the main rehabilitation operations reviewed

#	Agencies/utilities involved	Interventions	Period
1	Kabul:		
	KfW – World Bank/CAWSS	Repairs on Kabul Network. Phases I and II	2002–?
	ICRC – Spanish Red Cross/CAWSS	Rehabilitation and improvement of water supply in the north-west of Kabul	2002–2003
	ACF	Water and sanitation programme	2001–2005
2	Jaffna:		
	GTZ/JMC water services	Jaffna Rehabilitation Project	1997–2003
3	Monrovia:		
	European Union/LWSC	Essential repairs and support to LWSC	1996–2003
	European Union – World Bank/LWSC	Rehabilitation of Monrovia water distribution network and water distribution reform	2005–2006
	UNICEF	Support to water supply in Central Monrovia	2004–2006
	Oxfam	Water and sanitation project in Clara Town	2005–2006
4	Béni:		
	Solidarités – Aquassistance/REGIDESO	New water distribution network construction	2003–2005
5	Port-au-Prince:		
	GRET/CAMEP	Water supply for low-income neighbourhoods of Port-au-Prince	1995–2005

infrastructural works, a reform of CAWSS was planned. This reform encouraged CAWSS to have recourse to 'service providers' for water distribution (MUDH, 2005). These service providers were meant to be private companies and establishing one or several management contracts was a solution suggested by Beller-Kocks in order to achieve a better management of water distribution in Kabul.

During the same period, the ICRC, together with the Spanish Red Cross, implemented a similar project, albeit at a much smaller scale. It covered five areas of the city and consisted of the drilling and rehabilitation of boreholes, the construction of a new water reservoir and the rehabilitation of parts of the distribution network.

These two interventions focused mostly on areas served by the water network (the so-called 'planned areas'), whilst, in contrast, ACF focused specifically on 'unplanned areas' and worked largely independently from CAWSS. In 2003, ACF undertook a study in order to map vulnerability in

Kabul and decided to intervene in the poorest neighbourhoods, which are outside the areas served by the central water network. The organization drilled or rehabilitated boreholes in these areas and equipped them with handpumps. It also trained communities to effectively manage the operation and maintenance of the facilities.

Jaffna. Having sorted out emergency operations in Jaffna, GTZ sponsored the rehabilitation of the water distribution network. It started in December 1997 and lasted until 2001 (although GTZ support continued until 2003). This consisted mainly of the reconstruction or repairs of pumping stations, reservoirs, and water networks. GTZ retained project planning, recruitment of local and international experts, procurement of material and equipment, and monitoring and evaluation. JMC water services carried out all construction work (van Horen, 2002: 121).

Monrovia. In May 1996 the European Union funded the consulting firm Geoscience to carry out emergency support to LWSC. Its main tasks were to support water production and distribution as well as institutional strengthening. After the fall of Taylor's regime in 2003, the European Union decided to redefine the orientation of this assistance. Studies recommended supporting the introduction of the private sector in the management of Monrovia's water distribution network. It was therefore decided to divide Monrovia into concessions to be serviced by private companies or local user groups. This project was initiated in March 2005 by the German engineering firm 'Hydroplan'. The 2005 presidential election, however, brought considerable modifications of this plan. In February 2006, the new government was committed to an increased piped-water supply in Monrovia within six months. In order to fulfil this commitment, LWSC undertook major repairs on the network and on 26 July 2006, water reached areas of Central Monrovia after almost 15 years of interruption. The new LWSC management asked that, before implementing privatization, the World Bank, the European Union, and the government should support a major overhaul of the water network. A greater involvement of the community in the management of the concessions was also required. Six years later, the project continues.

Before the 2006 increased supply of piped water to the city, UNICEF was helping eight communities in Central Monrovia to manage the water they bought from tankers thus avoiding intermediary water sellers. In 2004, the organization donated a number of water storage facilities and water committees were organized.

Oxfam's intervention started in 2005 and focused on Clara Town, one of the most densely populated areas of Monrovia. It is a low-income area which is supplied with piped water from the water treatment plant. People obtain drinking water primarily from illegal vendors who are called 'water miners' because they have to dig holes in the ground or use existing manholes to make illegal connections to the water network since the pressure is too low to allow water to reach above ground level. The accumulation of surface water in these holes or manholes increases the threat of contamination in an area where environmental conditions are very poor.

The project, on the one hand, ensured that water delivery was hygienic and on the other helped communities get organized while obtaining the legalization of certain of their water vendors. Oxfam installed proper plumbing and storage tanks on water connections and obtained exclusive rights for vendors to sell water in their area.

Béni. The town of Béni, located near the border between the Kivu and Ituri regions, suffered from the effect of the armed conflicts that affected both regions. Between 1996 and 1999, equipment belonging to the water utility REGIDESO was looted. As a result, service deteriorated and 85 per cent of bills from commercial customers remained unpaid. From 2000, REGIDESO requested Solidarités to support the rehabilitation of the town's water network. The project actually started in 2003 and was completed in 2005. The project also involved the French agency Aquassistance (an organization offering technical assistance in the water sector).

By the end of the intervention, a new water treatment plant was built and an entirely new network of water kiosks set up. REGIDESO personnel were trained on how to run the new water treatment plant and were involved in the set-up of water committees in charge of managing the water kiosks (Neumann, 2006).

Port-au-Prince. Since 1995, GRET has been working on the improvement of water supply in a number of shantytowns of Port-au-Prince. What started as an emergency operation evolved into institutional development, both of community groups and of the water utility, CAMEP.

The programme aimed to extend the water distribution network to these shantytowns. It also worked with communities in order to enable them to manage water distribution and cost recovery in their neighbourhoods.

- In 1995 and 1996, GRET directly implemented works in the targeted shantytowns and supervised water committees.
- From 1997 to 1999, the responsibility of implementing works was progressively transferred to CAMEP, which dealt directly with water committees.
- From 2000, the role of GRET was limited to what the organization called 'social mediation' between communities and the water utility (Braïlovsky et al., 2000).

Findings

While a certain level of partnership between local water sector institutions and aid agencies always exists in interventions involving works on a water distribution network, the review of the case studies suggested that, in most cases, agencies' primary objectives remained focused on infrastructure.

Achieving sustainability through institutional development of the water utility has proved difficult and the research found little evidence of success, either in relatively small rehabilitation projects such as in Jaffna and Béni or in the large-scale water systems rehabilitation projects of Kabul and Monrovia, with important institutional development aspects. Moreover, the latter tend to target areas already served by a water distribution network and neglect a large proportion of the urban population, especially in the low-income areas. In contrast, relying solely on communities for the operation and maintenance of systems (such as in Kabul's 'unplanned areas' or in certain parts of Monrovia) may also fail to achieve sustainability, since it often depends on the presence of a few motivated community members.

The findings lead to the following conclusions:

- Partnerships between water sector institutions and aid agencies are frequent in rehabilitation/reconstruction but most of the interventions reviewed have shown little evidence of these partnerships contributing to sustainability.
- Large-scale rehabilitation projects are carried out in close collaboration with water utilities and encourage 'policy-driven' systems, i.e. systems regulated by an official institution. The research suggests that current strategies fail to effectively contribute to their institutional development. Instead, international financial institutions involved in the process prefer to encourage privatization of large portions of the service in order to substitute poorly performing utilities by supposedly more efficient private companies. Privatization in this environment is usually only viable in middle- and high-income neighbourhoods, which tend to already be served by a water network.
- Smaller-scale, community-based projects focus on low-income areas and have a limited interaction with water utilities. They reproduce mechanisms typical of the rural environment or of emergency response, thereby setting up 'needs-driven' systems, responding to immediate needs of the recipient population. Their outcomes tend to lack sustainability.

This rather negative assessment does not imply that partnerships are never justified. It only suggests that achieving sustainability and universal services through partnerships requires a paradigm shift. This would involve adopting a different, more balanced strategy that would encompass fostering the institutional development of the water utility and ensuring the consultation of consumers' communities. Most practitioners would agree with this but it is rarely put into practice in the field. Some elements explaining this situation are described in the following section.

Lessons to be learned

Combining skills

Maximizing the benefits of infrastructure rehabilitation entails working simultaneously on institutional development of the water utility and on social mobilization of communities. Achieving this goal requires diverse skills and collaboration between different types of organization.

Analysing how interventions were carried out suggests that these skills do exist among actors involved in rehabilitation projects. Commercial consulting firms are capable of engaging in institutional development of water utilities, albeit with unequal success. However, they rarely interact with consumer communities, often because their terms of reference do not require that they do so. In contrast, agencies involved in smaller-scale projects, in particular NGOs, often base their action on community participation. They are more prone to work on the social aspects of water projects but do not always consult water utilities. Differences exist in the ethical motivations, type of personnel, and agendas between them, which make collaboration especially difficult.

Interviews carried out on Kabul and Monrovia show that NGOs and consulting firms often work side by side, but with different methods, and little interaction. Resolving these differences requires that a coordinating body encourages or even imposes closer links between the various skills available. For that, a sufficiently strong leadership is indispensable.

There is no straightforward answer to how this leadership can be created. Ideally, this should be the task of governments and their public utilities. It is their responsibility to ensure that rehabilitation is carried out in a coordinated fashion. Unfortunately, government agencies are often too weak to play this prominent role. They may only carry such responsibility if donors encourage this change. It is therefore important to raise awareness among donors in order to ensure that rehabilitation programmes are designed to tackle both utility and community levels simultaneously and in a coordinated fashion.

Reconciling sustainability and universal service

Sustainability of urban services has three components: technological, financial, and institutional. Capacity building of the water utility contributes to technological sustainability by training technicians on how to run the service. Interventions tackling social aspects, including, among others, community consultation, contribute to institutional sustainability, which depends on communities relying on the service. Consumers' willingness to pay and affordability would in turn guarantee financial sustainability.

In most cases, the research pointed out a different reality. Often, institutional sustainability cannot be achieved because rehabilitation projects were found to intervene either exclusively at central level through water sector institutions, or in specific neighbourhoods with their respective communities. There were limited links between these two levels. Agencies working at central level usually aimed at restoring the situation prevailing 'before' the armed conflict, in which the utility distributed water through private connections to a limited number of consumers. Kabul is a good example: a master plan designed in 1974 was taken as the basis for the 2003 rehabilitation of the water distribution network despite the considerable changes induced by war.

After years of conflict and massive population displacements, cities such as Kabul, Monrovia, and many others changed dramatically. Rehabilitation projects must adapt to the new state of the city, rather than trying to reproduce conditions from the past.

For that, working with communities is essential in order to understand and quantify their needs. For instance, in certain neighbourhoods, in general the richest, privatizing water distribution may be beneficial. In others, often the poorest, a different model, such as community management, may be the answer. In Monrovia, the situation found suggested that the most realistic solution would have been to work on the 'legalization' of the multitude of private vendors who took over most of municipal water supply. To a certain extent, Oxfam tried to follow that path in Clara Town.

Agencies working at neighbourhood level with communities may contribute to sustainability if they act as intermediaries between the water utility and consumers. In this way, mechanisms of accountability can be established, thereby giving a 'voice' to the consumers on how water services are delivered in their area.

Building confidence in institutions

Water sector institutions are sometimes assigned advisers in order to foster their institutional development. These advisers are usually staff employed by commercial consulting firms managing large-scale rehabilitation projects. Both in Kabul and Monrovia the research found considerable mistrust between these firms and the staff of the water utility whose capacity they are meant to strengthen. Confronted with the apparently irresolvable problem of encouraging reforms in order to restore efficiency and profitability to the water utility in a relatively short timeframe, commercial consulting firms may recommend privatization, however improbable, as a possible solution.

Reconstruction money gives aid agencies more power and an opportunity of influencing strategies with newly established governments more willing to break with the past and undertake reforms. In these conditions, privatization would be missing a crucial opportunity or demonstrate a lack of interest from aid agencies for institutional development of the water utility. Changes within LWSC in Monrovia, which took place in 2006 and led to the restoration of water supply in areas after many years, show that, in certain cases, untapped resources may exist within local institutions. Of course, this is largely dependent on the political will of local governments.

Building confidence between water utilities and aid agencies is also important when working with communities. Aid agencies may help in re-establishing a bond existing between certain communities and public services. These communities are usually the most vulnerable and often live in the peri-urban areas. Whilst gaining access to municipal services, they also regain the status of citizen, from which they were previously excluded. This was a major achievement of GRET's project in Port-au-Prince. Water utilities may be changed through this process and adopt a 'customer orientation'; in other words, a policy aiming to establishing a genuine dialogue with existing and potential customers.

About the author

Jean-François Pinera (jfpinera@gmail.com) is a water engineer, recently re turned from Haiti and currently working for the International Committee of the Red Cross on relief and rehabilitation projects similar to those mentioned Red Cross on relief and rehabilitation projects similar to those mentioned comments on this article.

References

Anand, P.B. (2005) *Getting Infrastructure Priorities Right in Post Conflict Reconstruction*, Research Paper Ref. 2005/42, United Nations University/World Institute for Development Economics Research, Helsinki.

Braïlovsky, A., Boisgallais, A. and Paquot, E. (2000) *Coopérer Aujourd'hui: Intermédiation sociale et construction institutionnelle: démarches du programme d'approvisionnement en eau des quartiers populaires de Port-au-Prince en Haïti*, Ref. 15, Groupe de Recherche et d'Echange Technologique, Paris.

Brinkhof, T. (2011) *City Population* [website], <http://www.citypopulation.de> [accessed August 2011].

Buchanan-Smith, M. and Maxwell, S. (1994) 'Linking relief and development: An introduction and overview', *IDS bulletin* 25(4): 2–16.

Duffield, M. (1994) 'Complex emergencies and the crisis of developmentalism', *IDS bulletin* 25(4): 37–45.

Hodgson, R. and Oppliger, A. (1998) 'After the battle of Grozny', in ICRC (ed.), *Forum, 1: War and Water*, pp. 66-71, International Committee of the Red Cross, Geneva.

ICRC (2006) *Operational Update: Haiti: A Year and a Half's Work in Cité Soleil*, Ref. 06/4, International Committee of the Red Cross, Geneva.

Matthieussent, S. and Carlier, R. (2004) 'Le cas de l'approvisionnement en eau potable des quartiers défavorisés de Port-au-Prince. Document de travail', in Groupe de Recherche et d'Echange Technologique (ed.), *Séminaires sur les politiques publiques de lutte contre la pauvreté et les inégalités, 17/11/04*, Reseau Impact – Politique Africaine, Paris.

MUDH (2005) *Urban Water Supply and Sewerage Sector Institutional Development Plan*, Ministry of Urban Development and Housing, Islamic Republic of Afghanistan, Kabul.

Murshed, S.M. (2002) 'Conflict, civil war and underdevelopment: An introduction', *Peace Research Abstracts* 40(4): 387–93.

Neumann, B. (2006) 'Les effets vertueux des fontaines de Béni', *L'Expansion* 710: 72–75.

Ockelford, J. (1993) 'How do we work with host government and other NGOs for the good of the refugees (Workshop 3). Discussion paper: Coordination of emergency relief in Liberia', in B. Reed (ed.), *Technical Support for Refugees. Proceedings of the 1991 International Conference. 17-18 December 1991*, pp. 27-39, Water Engineering and Development Centre, Loughborough University, Loughborough, UK.

Pinera, J. and Reed, R.A. (2007) 'Maximizing aid benefits after urban disasters through partnerships with local water sector utilities', *Disasters Prevention and Management* 16(3): 401–11.

Slaymaker, T., Christiansen, K. and Hemming, I. (2005) *Community-based Approaches and Service Delivery: Issues and Options in Difficult Environments and Partnerships*, Overseas Development Institute, London.

Smillie, I. (2001) 'Capacity building and the humanitarian enterprise', in Ian Smillie (ed.), *Patronage and Partnership*, pp. 7–23, Kumarian Press, Bloomfield, CT.

Solidarités (1998) *Programme d'aide d'urgence à Kaboul. Eau et Assainissement. Rapport final*. Ref. ECHO/AFG/210/1998/01023, Solidarités, Paris.

Themnér, L. and Wallensteen, P. (2011) 'Armed conflict, 1946–2010', *Journal of Peace Research* 48(4): 525–36.

United Nations Population Division (2009) *World Urbanization Prospects: The 2009 Revision* [website], UN Department of Economic and Social Affairs <http://esa.un.org/unpd/wup/index.htm> [accessed August 2011].

van Horen, B. (2002) 'Planning for institutional capacity building in war-torn areas: The case of Jaffna, Sri Lanka', *Habitat International* 26(1): 113–28.

CHAPTER 10
Sanitation for all! Free of cost in emergencies

Marco Visser

Abstract

Food and clean water are provided for free in refugee camps, so why are refugees expected to provide public sanitation facilities themselves? Refugees often have to contribute labour and materials in constructing these facilities just at a time when they are most exhausted or traumatized. Marco Visser argues that sanitation should be provided free in these situations.

Early 2010, Haiti was struck by a catastrophic earthquake, followed by a 'tsunami' of humanitarian aid. Despite the massive numbers of aid agencies and multimillion dollars of aid money being pumped into the county, a cholera epidemic broke out and quickly spread as from October that same year. This cholera outbreak once again demonstrates that what seems to be the case in development aid – the fact that 'water is hot, sanitation is not' – also applies to emergency relief. The outbreak would never have been this widespread if the sanitary conditions in the camps had been of a certain minimum standard.

Provision of safe drinking water is, rightfully so, the first priority in an emergency situation such as the consequence of a man-made or natural disaster. People simply don't survive without drinking water. So, it is not surprising that water supply receives a lot of attention and resources in such a situation. Water supply is also more 'mediagenic' than sanitation. Who wouldn't rather boast about that smart looking machine making crystal-clear drinking water from a murky pool than about a squatting field? Unfortunately, this results in sanitation receiving a lot less attention and consequently fewer resources.

Those few aid agencies that are engaged in sanitation activities in camps often swear by a development approach, whereby participation, community involvement, ownership, and sustainability is considered imperative. This means that refugees and internally displaced persons (IDPs), often traumatized and trying hard to survive, are nearly always expected to assist in the construction of sanitary facilities, for example by digging pits or providing building materials, without any form of compensation, since the facilities are for their benefit. And as they are using the facilities, they surely will have to maintain them, again for free.

http://dx.doi.org/10.3362/9781780448831.010

This would be acceptable, if it were private or household facilities. But if one has to share the latrine with 50 or more other users, this becomes another matter, especially when these other users, despite being neighbours in the camp, are complete strangers to one another. Communities and families may well have separated in the course of the disaster, and camps do not necessarily form tight 'natural communities'.

So, whereas water often remains available for free for as long as is needed, sanitation seems to come with a price. It seems that different rules of engagement apply for sanitation in emergencies. This is not just odd and inconsistent, but moreover unfortunate and wrong, as sanitation in any situation is – at least – as important as water supply in preventing and controlling communicable disease.

Though the debate continues about the effects of water supply versus sanitation, quantity versus quality and community supply versus household connections, there is no doubt that the need for sanitation in emergencies is even more prominent than in a non-emergency situation. This is for a number of reasons. First of all, people affected have often fled their homes and been travelling for a substantial time. Weak and exhausted after days, sometimes weeks of fleeing without food, drink, and shelter, has made them extremely vulnerable and susceptible to all kinds of disease. When finally settling down in a public building, a makeshift or a more organized camp, the chances are that those people are still without some form of shelter for the first few days and still exposed to the rain, cold or heat, and disease-transmitting insects. Often, camps are (to be) sited in the least habitable locations, either extremely arid or – at the other extreme – swampy and infested with mosquitoes. Lastly, in the area where the refugees settle there may be certain diseases prevalent that do not exist in their place of origin. This means no resistance to those diseases.

This all means that in an emergency the chance of contracting a disease is many times higher than pre-emergency. So, if on top of this the sanitary conditions in the camp are poor – which is often the case – the chance of falling ill basically turns to certainty. And with an extremely high population density, the disease spreads easier, faster, and wider, eventually turning into an uncontrollable outbreak.

Sanitation should therefore receive the same amount of attention and resources – if not more – than water supply in emergencies. As top priority in any emergency, sufficient, safe, and high quality facilities should be provided. Provided for free. There should be no 'forced voluntarism' demanded from the affected population. Aside from the fact that people may be traumatized and have other priorities, those unable to participate are also likely to be excluded. They include child-headed households, elderly and the physically and mentally disabled, who in an emergency can form a large proportion of the population.

Whereas it is totally accepted that water, food, and medical services are provided for free in an emergency, providing sanitation services for free seems to be anathema. The consequence is that in nearly every emergency and every camp the sanitary conditions are appalling. To tackle this, aid agencies should be willing to provide sanitation facilities for free and pay for the labour and materials required. In this way, they also provide a welcome income for the affected community to be used for example for purchasing extra food supplies, soap, and other necessities.

In a sense, it is rather surprising that aid agencies tend to revert to development approaches for emergency relief sanitation interventions. Every WASH intervention should comprise 'hardware' and 'software' components and it is a fact that the latter is usually the hardest. Technically, everything is possible, but when it comes to behaviour change and adaptation – the 'software' aspects – it is something else. To that effect, an emergency should be rather simple, as in this case one could to a certain extent ignore the 'software'. Old habits, however, unfortunately seem to die hard.

One more advantage of providing sufficient, safe, and clean sanitation free of cost in emergencies only reveals itself post-emergency, when the affected population has returned or relocated. Marketing sanitation has proved itself as one of the most successful methods of increasing the number of people with access to improved sanitation. As with any product, sales, or in this case the uptake, grow with demand. And demand grows when the product is associated positively. So when people have experienced the sanitation facilities in the camp in a positive way, meaning they were appropriate, comfortable, and clean, their demand for such facilities post-emergency will be high. If, on the other hand, they have only had dirty, smelly, and insect-ridden facilities at their disposal, they are unlikely to want such a facility post-emergency.

About the author

Marco Visser (info@washforlife.nl) is a private consultant with extensive experience in emergency WASH, Public Health and Environmental Engineering. He is founder and owner of WASH for life (www.washforlife.nl).

CHAPTER 11
Conclusions

Richard C. Carter

This book provides some context and current practical reflections on how to do WASH better in response to emergencies. It is not intended to be comprehensive in its scope, but it addresses various important contextual issues and key aspects of water, sanitation and hygiene in emergencies. The main chapters have provided some real and recent examples of the difficulties of meeting people's WASH needs in emergencies, but they have all gone further with pertinent and practical recommendations for practitioners and aid organizations. If action is taken on even a few of these recommendations, progress will be made.

As overall editor, my own personal recommendations at the end of this book are first to the practitioners and professionals who bring their commitment and dedication to bear on some very difficult situations:

- try as hard as you can and as often as you can to document and publish the tacit knowledge which you have in such abundance – and which others need to benefit from. I believe this book shows the benefits of doing that;
- build links between those who specialize in so-called humanitarian response and those whose expertise is in long-term development; identify differences of approach and work to resolve these in imaginative new ways;
- collaborate whenever possible with researchers, who can help to systematize your knowledge, and with knowledge brokers, who can help to disseminate it.

And to the aid agencies:

- listen to and be guided by humanitarian and development field workers as you determine your organizations' evolving policy and strategy;
- commit resources to support linkages between field workers, researchers, knowledge brokers and other professionals as we all strive to do WASH better in emergencies.

Lightning Source UK Ltd.
Milton Keynes UK
UKHW02f1950040718
325226UK00003B/157/P